Allergies

Disease in Disguise

Allergies

Disease in Disguise

How to heal your allergic condition permanently and naturally

Carolee Bateson-Koch DC ND

Foreword by Lendon H. Smith MD

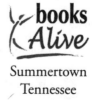

books
Alive

Summertown
Tennessee

Cover Design: Ivan A. de Lorenzana, Scott Yavis, *alive* Publishing Group Inc.
Cover Photo: Digital Stock

Note to Readers:
The information in this book is for educational purposes only. It is not in-
tended, and should not be considered, as a replacement for consultation, di-
agnosis or treatment by a duly licensed health practitioner.

Published by **Books Alive**
a division of Book Publishing Company
PO Box 99
Summertown, TN 38483
(888) 260-8458   www.bookpubco.com

Printed in the United States of America

16 15 14 13 12   12 13 14 15 16

ISBN 978-1-55312-040-7
    The Library of Congress has already cataloged an earlier printing under
the publisher name "Alive Books" as follows:
    Library of Congress Cataloging-in-Publication Data
    Bateson-Koch, Carolee, 1942-
    Allergies, disease in disguise : how to heal your allergic condition perma-
nently and naturally / Carolee Bateson-Koch ; foreword by Lendon H. Smith.
        p. cm.
    Includes bibliographical references and index.
    ISBN 978-1-55312-040-7 (alk. paper)
    1. Allergy--Popular works. 2. Allergy--Alternative treatment. 3. Natur-
opathy. I. Title.
    RC585.B38 2008
    616.97--dc22   2008015401

Books Alive is a member of Green Press Initiative. We chose to print this title on
paper with postconsumer recycled content, processed without chlorine, which
saved the following natural resources:

1,333 pounds of solid waste   46 trees
18 million BTU of net energy 21,028 gallons of water
4,663 pounds of greenhouse gases

For more information, visit www.greenpressinitiative.org.
Savings calculations thanks to the Environmental Defense Paper Calculator,
www.edf.org/papercalculator.

*Dedicated in memory to
my husband Dr. Helmut G. Koch
whose dynamic energy and dedication to healing
others will always be remembered.*

Contents

Contents

List of Figures

Foreword

About twenty years ago I began to realize that allergies were causing more than sneezing, wheezing and itching. The parents of my patients were telling me about odd symptoms for which there were no explanations. Emmy got a headache after eating wheat, or Jonathan became hyper if he had orange juice. At first I scoffed at these anecdotal observations because I thought the mothers were trying to avoid blame for some psychological maladjustment. Then when my own children began to have odd symptoms that defied a reasonable explanation, I began to believe these reports from many, many patients.

Allergies seemed to be an explanation, so I joined the American College of Allergists. At a meeting I attended in 1970, I was not too surprised to find that there was a schism in the ranks of the members. A new group, the food sensitivity believers, was just forming at that meeting. Dr. James Breneman was the leader of these "radicals." He cited some studies done on bed-wetting that showed that the lining of the bladder in most bed-wetters was speckled with eosinophils, a clear sign of allergy. (That made me feel good because I had been a bed-wetter as a boy and had a son with the problem, which turned out to be a milk sensitivity. No milk, no wet bed. The explanation from psychiatrists was that the child hated the mother and emptied his bladder on the bed – sub-consciously meaning mom.)

In general, however, the group realized they were on shaky ground because there was no test that could clearly distinguish between patients with positive RAST or skin tests and patients with food sensitivities. A reliable, valid, reproducible test would take the anecdotes out of the old wives' category and put food sensitivities into a clinically useful setting. Until recently the only method of diagnosing these food reactions was to present symptoms to a doctor who happens to believe in the reliability of the patient. For example: "After I eat beef (or corn, cheese, soy, peanuts, shellfish, MSG, aspartame, etc.), I feel weak (mean, get a headache, cramps, diarrhea, bloody nose, etc.)." Doctor's response is, "don't eat those things." So much for science in the clinical setting. Doctors are loath to believe that a patient's list of symptoms has any validity without some blood test, X-ray, or palpable lump. When I found food sensitivities in myself and my family, that explained mood swings, hyperactivity, bedwetting, migraines and arthritis, it was easy to find similar reactions in my patients.

At that meeting 22 years ago I learned two things: that 80% of people with food sensitivities have hypoglycemia, and that food sensitivities cannot do everything, but they can do anything. The standard, traditional allergists are careful to point out that the RAST (Radioallergosorbent Test) or the skin prick test using extracts, diagnoses real allergies. The treatment is to give injections of these antigen-containing extracts in gradually increasing doses to block the allergic reaction.

I thought sugar would be the villain in the hyperactivity scenario, but although that food was part of the picture, it was milk, corn, additives, salicylates, and more importantly, anything the person liked (and craved) that caused of the symptoms. About 60% of my hyperactive patients had mood swings and restless behavior if they drank milk. They loved milk. I did tests on these children and discovered they were all low in calcium. No wonder they craved the stuff; they needed the calcium. Apparently, however, no matter how much they drank, it was not absorbed because the intestinal lining cells rejected it. Calcium from other foods plus calcium supplements was necessary to provide helpful therapy for their restless behavior.

I have been delighted with this reassuring, informative, scientifically validated book. It gives me a warm feeling to find a kindred therapist in Dr. Carolee Bateson-Koch. I believe everyone suffers from some food sensitivity. The clues are in this book. Before a person runs off to the psychiatrist because the doctor can find nothing wrong, I recommend he or she read this book. The methods outlined in this book should give some relief. Most readers will discover that they are not hypochondriacs or emotional cripples. They are normal human beings forced to breathe polluted air, eat processed food and drink contaminated water.

In summary, the body should be so healthy that digestion will break the ingested foods down into their basic, non-allergic amino acids, fatty acids and simple carbohydrates. It makes sense then, to try to balance the pH of the body, take in nutrient-adequate foods and maintain a low-stress lifestyle. If problems persist, digestive enzyme supplements should help the body maintain homeostasis. We aim for not just health, but for a robust zest for living.

Lendon H. Smith, MD

Lendon H. Smith, MD is the author of:
Happiness is a Healthy Life, Feed Yourself Right, Feed Your Kids Right, Foods for Healthy Kids, Dr. Lendon Smith's Low Stress Diet, Clinical Guide to the Use of Vitamin C and *Hyper Kids.*

Preface

Over my 33 years in practice as a doctor of chiropractic and naturopathy, it became apparent to me that some other factor was underlying many of the musculoskeletal conditions that I was treating. In searching for answers, I became aware of the involvement of allergy, not only in musculoskeletal conditions, but in many other conditions as well. Further research confirmed my suspicion that allergy is a serious disorder with far-reaching effects – it is much more than just a runny nose. The life-long work of doctors such as Randolph, Rowe, Breneman and Crook lends validity to this new and broader concept of allergy.

The incidence of allergies is on the rise. In the United States 40 to 50 million people, or one-in-five adults and children, suffer from allergies. Of these people, 74% report that their allergies interfere with their work and social lives. The most popular methods of fighting allergy, antihistamines, and decongestants; avoiding dust, smoke, pets, perfume and mold; purifying the air; have for the most part, been ineffective. Thousands of people with allergic manifestations are going untreated because the true cause of their symptoms is unrecognized.

I further believe that it is just as important for a doctor to teach wellness as it is to make health recommendations. People need to understand and should have the information to understand whatever therapy they choose. Their decisions should be informed decisions. The need for real help for allergic disorders is overwhelming.

Allergies, Disease in Disguise answers that need. It goes beyond telling the reader how to relieve, manage, control or attack allergies; it offers sound, scientific advice and a straightforward method for overcoming allergies.

Allergies, Disease in Disguise...

Informs the reader, in simple terms, how common health problems are actually allergic diseases.

Identifies the three most common overlooked conditions that lead to allergic disorders.

Imparts the secret of food allergy.

Presents an updated, fresh perspective on the process of digestion and how it relates to allergy.

Explains enzyme therapy – a safe, non-toxic treatment based on scientific research and clinical experience.

Describes six common allergic conditions of children and what to do about them.

Explores a new allergic phenomenon, electromagnetic hypersensitivity syndrome, which affects thousands of people worldwide.

Many times, at the end of a television or radio interview, the announcer asks me the question, "What message would you like to leave our listeners with today?" It is this. You can get well from allergy. Allergy is not a permanent condition that you must learn to live with, as some authorities would have you believe. Not only can you heal your allergies; it is not as difficult as you might think.

Many thanks to:

My mother, Dr. Virginia Coffman,
for her encouragement, stimulating questions,
helpful suggestions and the hard work of proofreading.

My husband, Dr. Helmut Koch,
for his support, assistance and willingness to discuss ideas.
His graciousness was appreciated when time for writing this
book interfered with personal and professional schedules.

Gisela Temmel, managing editor at Alive Books,
for her editing skills, helpful advice, guidance and
enthusiasm for this book.

Help for a Mysterious, Obscure Disorder

Leona's Success Story as Told by her Mother

At birth, Leona was a beautiful, healthy 8-lb. 11-oz. baby girl. At an early age, she had a tendency to develop ear infections and as time went on, she frequently had hearing loss due to fluid in her ears. I took her to her doctor on a regular basis, but I did not elect to put in ear tubes, as I was afraid that they might cause hearing loss in Leona's later years. When Leona was two or three, I discovered that a drink of milk before a car trip would always cause her to vomit approximately 30 miles from home. Leona also complained a great deal about aching legs and a "sore belly." As the years rolled by, Leona had bouts of extremely runny noses, coupled with bad colds that required two or three boxes of tissue a day. When Leona was around ten years old, I suspected milk to be causing her problems so I took her off milk completely. It was like magic! No more sore legs ("growing pains"), no runny nose and no more "sore belly" like before when she had eaten cereal with milk in the morning. These symptoms only reoccurred after Leona cheated and ate or drank dairy products.

However, Leona still had other complaints such as occasional pains in her abdominal area, vaguely likened to appendicitis. In grade 5, Leona almost fainted in school but recovered quickly. While playing hockey, she would occasionally get weak and have to leave the game. At swimming class Leona would often feel unwell, but was still able to earn her Bronze Medallion and Bronze Cross when she was

14. At this point, I took her to two different doctors but nothing was ever found.

It was about this time that I discovered that food would perk her up. Leona was twelve when we made a day excursion to the zoo. After walking two or three miles, Leona became very weak and fatigued and was unable to walk any further. I was about to find a ride back to our vehicle but remembered that sweets seemed to give her energy so I bought a sweet orange drink. Leona recovered quickly and was able to walk back.

Leona had always been very hard to get to sleep. Even as a baby, she slept the bare minimum. As she grew older, she would lie awake in bed waiting for sleep to come. It was not unusual to hear her up at one, two or even three in the morning looking for a snack. Schoolwork was always a struggle, although Leona did well. In order to get good marks, hours and hours of work and study were required. Leona complained of major difficulty concentrating. She would read a textbook but then did not know what she had read. She also complained that the words ""jumped around"" and she would often lose her place on the page while reading. Leona always had crusty eyelids and her ears were often very sensitive to sound.

As Leona matured, she had more fainting spells and incidents of severe abdominal pain and headaches. She frequently did not feel good and exhibited unreasonable angry outbursts and mood swings. Her symptoms became more severe, including attacks of intense abdominal pain, ravenous hunger and craving for sugar. Low blood sugar (hypoglycemia) was now suspected and Leona's doctor put her on a hypoglycemia diet. The low sugar content of the diet helped her mood swings and insomnia but when I gave her the high protein (lots of eggs and peanut butter sandwiches) she began to deteriorate and got much worse than ever. (Leona had previously decided to eliminate meat, poultry and fish from her diet).

At this point the intense abdominal pain was frequent; she was always ravenous, and her energy level was way down. Leona had been very athletic but now she had to stop playing hockey, a sport she had enjoyed for six years. More often than not, she was pale and "did not feel good," had sensitive ears, smelly feet, and drowsy-looking eyes.

Leona was now missing a lot of school so her doctor got her an appointment with a specialist. After four days of extensive tests, exams and consultations including an unnecessary psychiatric exam (I knew she was physically sick, not imagining illness), the doctors came to the conclusion that there was nothing they could find wrong with her physically or mentally.

That same day, Leona was too tired to climb a flight of stairs without resting. So now with all conventional medical causes ruled out and the condition still existing, we went to see a nutritionist. The nutritionist advised us to eliminate wheat, egg yolks, yeast, sugar and dairy products from Leona's diet. (Dairy products had already been eliminated). The nutritionist also advised Leona to take a multiple vitamin, calcium, magnesium and flaxseed oil.

Three days later, Leona was well on the road to recovery. A great deal of her symptoms had disappeared. Leona followed the diet rigidly for six weeks, which included her exam time at school. In this set of exams, her marks improved dramatically; some subjects as much as 40 points. After exams were over, Leona was feeling so good (back to playing hockey), she thought that it would not hurt to cheat on her diet. She had a McDonald's apple turnover, a bar, and some cheese. Two days later she had a runny nose, tonsillitis with a temperature of 103.6° F and intense stomach pains. Leona learned the consequences of her experience and after that, stayed on her diet very rigidly except for one or two incidents of cheating and some accidental eating of forbidden foods.

We learned that even small amounts of refined sugar would cause intense abdominal pain two days later and small amounts of wheat caused intestinal distress and dairy products caused abdominal discomfort, aching legs and nose, ear and throat problems. Cigarette smoke also produced major symptoms of discomfort.

By now, we knew for sure that Leona felt "awesome" when she stayed off wheat, sugar, yeast, egg yolk, and dairy products. She was much more pleasant to have around. We knew that when she cheated on her diet she felt terrible and couldn't go to school or play hockey. It then took 2 to 4 days to recover, as she was lethargic and easily tired. On these interim days, Leona would go to the hockey rink, suit up,

3

play a few shifts and have to take off her gear. She even had to lie down on the bench of the dressing room. Leona had the desire to keep going, and pushed herself to the limit, but had to give in anyway.

Outwardly, at age 15, Leona looked reasonably well but she was always uncomfortable and fatigued. As she described it, each day she would get up, pull herself together, go to school and try to act well and happy, but when she came home she would fall apart. In class she found staying awake her main concern. Her teachers were tolerant and understanding and allowed her to eat frequent snacks, as she needed them. Her classmates accepted her weird food habits without teasing or ridicule and she had no social problems at school and she still fit in despite her health problems.

Although Leona was conscientious and cooperative about her diet and it had originally helped, she became more and more sensitive to foods so that no matter how hard we tried, if she accidentally consumed food containing perhaps only minute quantities of allergens, it was enough for her to react severely.

I realized at that point that the diet was only a stopgap measure that wasn't going to work very well for much longer. I continued to read everything I could get my hands on concerning allergy or food intolerance.

We have a family history of allergy. Hives would break out when my father ate strawberries and honey. My mother was sensitive to perfume and other scents. She was also sensitive to dairy products. One of my sons gets stuffed up and has nose bleeds when exposed to feathers and newly cut grass and close contact with cats causes his eyes to swell. He also can't seem to do without milk. One of my daughters is sensitive to milk and another daughter gets huge hives that we think are caused by a new scented detergent. I also have a maternal aunt with celiac disease.

I knew that it was up to me to find someone who would help Leona since the team of specialists at the Children's Hospital had found nothing wrong and she was certainly still very ill. I searched for names and addresses of health care professionals who practiced holistic medicine. I wrote up a case history and sent this off along with a picture of my five children and a cover letter asking for help and referrals. The response was excellent and many different names and remedies were sent to me.

It was about this time that I picked up Dr. Bateson-Koch's book *Allergies: Disease in Disguise* at the health food store. I immediately read the book cover-to-cover and was so excited that I called other people I knew who were interested in this subject. I reread the book and decided I had to talk to Dr. Bateson-Koch. After some detective work I found her phone number and spoke with her secretary who was very encouraging and our conversation left me with the feeling that Leona had to see Dr. Bateson-Koch. I mailed out Leona's medical records and her case history to Dr. Bateson-Koch. She called me back in early May 1994, and I was very impressed and she told me that she would see Leona. I was now receiving many letters and opinions on how to help Leona from the many good doctors who answered my letters. I compared treatment and methods used to help problems such as ours and I found Dr. Bateson-Koch's ideas made the most sense. She offered what I was looking for, to fix the problem where it started and not to simply mask the symptoms. I felt there was an underlying reason for Leona's sickness; a basic breakdown that caused all her problems. I felt Dr. Bateson-Koch was genuine. I did some more research and I found out from other doctors who were familiar with her that she was very sincere and dedicated and well worth going to see. That was all it took, so I made an appointment for Leona on June 23 and on May 26 I sealed it all when I bought two airplane tickets.

In the interval and acting on some ideas posed by Dr. Bateson-Koch, I had some more medical tests done to help diagnose Leona's problem. A blood test called Red Blood Cell Mineral Analysis was performed that showed that Leona's blood was low in calcium and magnesium. Leona was given a calcium-magnesium IV drip that was the first one ever done at our local hospital. The doctor also arranged for me to get a diagnostic stool analysis test for parasites, which turned out to be another first in our area.

While my search for a doctor had gone on, Leona had been feeling reasonably well and in February 1994, was having reactions only every week and a half or so. However, as time went by, the reactions

5

became closer and closer together. No matter how strictly she followed her diet it seemed that she would inadvertently ingest some food that would cause great discomfort. To illustrate my point, I'd like to mention a few incidents. On a ski trip she bought a bottle of "pure" juice and drank it without reading the ingredients on the label. It contained sugar and two days later at a dance she paid dearly. I had to come get her and found her crying with pain. With help, I got her out to our van and when we got home I somehow dragged her up the steps and into the house where she collapsed on the floor in a fetal position, crying many tears. These extreme reactions lasted about 45 minutes to an hour. The next day Leona would be too wiped out to go to school and for the next 3 to 4 days she would be very fatigued and experienced abdominal discomfort. Her eyes would only be part way open and the day before a reaction she would be very unreasonable and angry.

We are Catholic and Leona could not even take communion (the host is wheat). If she did take the host she would be fatigued and lethargic for about a day after taking it.

These reactions were now being triggered by smaller and smaller amounts of irritant and were happening so often they were overlapping. By the end of May, Leona's energy level was very low. She didn't go swimming with her friends when they went for the first swim of the year in June. She couldn't even go to the mall shopping with me. She would get so tired she would stay home. (Inability to shop is a real sign of trouble in a teenager). In school she was very tired and I would often have to take her home. After a day a school she would fall asleep on the couch in the midst of the noise and activities of four children. During June, Leona studied for her exams the best she could and wrote about half of them but she became too sick and tired to finish the rest of them. Her medical doctor gave her an excuse and she got her Grade 9 on the work she had already completed.

Leona was always ravenous and she ate constantly but she couldn't be filled. Then a very alarming incident happened. Leona's food was not being processed and began passing through her whole! Pancakes, muffins, raisins, carrots, oatmeal were all still recognizable in her stool. This scared me the most. I knew it meant major digestive problems. I now thanked God for my airplane tickets that I had bought.

I would like to mention the mental stress that an obscure condition such as Leona's can put on a family. First there was always doubt by some as to how sick she really was – the hospital tests said she was okay, didn't they? In this case, the appearance of good health was a problem. Even my best friends said, "But she sure looks good." Some doctors seemed to think Leona was just lazy. To compound all this there was the problem created by sugar. Sugar turned her into a belligerent, angry girl. It was sometimes hard to sympathize with someone so unreasonable even when I knew it was the sugar talking. It's hard to explain to others and myself that Leona couldn't help being this way; it wasn't her fault. She was as prickly as a cactus. Sugar made her a monster. The other children (at home) called her "the dragon" when she got up in the morning. No one dared speak to her or look at her for fear of an angry outburst. When a child is uncooperative, sullen, cranky and given to unreasonable rages she does not get as much sympathy or understanding as is due her. There were times I wondered where I went wrong in her upbringing, but when I looked at everything in perspective, I realized she was good inside but tormented by her illness, for I could see no reason for her actions.

In addition, there were all the extra expenses involved in the preparation of two types of meals every day. I also had to do all our own baking to avoid any sugar as well as working full time. I often wondered if would we ever have a normal life?

As I researched and talked to people I found others who suffered as Leona did. In early June when Leona was down pretty low I took her to see a new friend who has the same symptoms as Leona. They talked for a few hours and she felt relieved and not so alone.

All through this ordeal Leona never despaired or even mentioned the possibility of never getting better. She believed, as I told her that no matter what, I wouldn't stop searching until she was better.

On June 22 we left our home province to fly across Canada to see Dr. Bateson-Koch. We were met at the airport by Dr. Bateson-Koch. I thought this was a very warm gesture. The next day, Dr. Bateson-Koch examined Leona and I was amazed by her different approach but I felt very secure that this was the kind of medicine I wanted for my daughter. Dr. Bateson-Koch was skilled, confident and competent. My spirits rose and I felt a great weight being lifted off my shoulders. After a great deal of testing, Dr. Bateson-Koch gave Leona a program to follow for the next six weeks that included a diet specifically designed for Leona, vitamins and minerals, herbs, and enzymes. She was also given a list of foods to avoid. Leona was instructed to drink a lot of pure water. On the second day Leona felt a bit sick, which happens sometimes when toxins leave the body. Dr. Bateson-Koch has an excellent bedside manner and makes her patients feel important, comfortable and at ease. From that day on I was able to see Leona gradually become the girl she had the potential of being. She fewer reactions that were less and less severe. Her energy level shot up.

We left for home on June 30. I knew Leona was better but I wondered if it would last, and how much better she would be in a month or two, especially when we reintroduced the offending foods. From July first to the first of August, Leona had only one small reaction. It was the day she returned home and she had eaten Italian dressing at the airport. The reaction was about 1/3 as severe as usual. From then on she was reaction-free. Her energy and strength rebounded and her energy level was that of a normal athletic child. She was off the couch and down to the beach the rest of the summer. She was able to help around the house and her personality was much improved. Gone was the unreasonable girl. Dr. Bateson-Koch gave me back a nice understanding girl who now would take time to talk to me in a civilized manner. The doors stopped slamming and the sibling battles were way down. Just like a caterpillar she emerged from her illness as a butterfly, a smiling happy girl who I always knew was locked inside a sick body for too long.

By the second week of August we were up to test time; it was time to reintroduce some of the offending foods, the foods that had originally caused adverse reactions. Leona started with communion and no reaction happened; then biscuit and onto toast. No problem. Then came the big test - pizza. No reaction at all! Wonderful! She ate a large pizza with no problem. She took extra enzymes, of course.

This was the day the sun broke through. I was elated. Then, Leona, against my better judgement, ate cheese almost every day. Before long her legs began to ache. That was the sign for her to eat cheese only occasionally. One day she felt very brave and had a bit of brown sugar. That didn't work out well (not as severe as usual but uncomfortable) so she learned to leave sugar alone. Maple syrup seemed OK but we thought honey was not good, as it gave her an uncomfortable reaction in September. Many symptoms were really gone; it was almost too good to comprehend.

Leona's Before and After Symptoms:
Stomach and intestines:
> **Before:** Bloated, discomfort, pain, poor digestion, food going through whole. Had to wear loose-fitting clothes around her waist.
>
> **After:** No bloating, pain or discomfort. Good digestion and normal bowel action. Leona can now fit into her old jeans even if the legs are too short. She does not have a distended abdomen.

Nose:
> **Before:** Very runny and stuffed with post nasal drip.
>
> **After:** Almost all stopped. No mucus in the mouth in the morning.

Ears:
> **Before:** Ringing, fluid in ears, earaches.
>
> **After:** Ears are clear, with no fluid or ringing or sensitivity.

Eyes
> **Before:** Heavy-lidded eyes; blue circles under her eyes.
>
> **After:** Bright-eyes, circles no longer noticeable.

Eyelids:
> **Before:** Crusty; could not keep fully open.
>
> **After:** No symptoms.

Sleeping:
> **Before:** Leona was up until all hours of the night and feeling very hungry. She would eat almost anything. She had problems resting at night and it would be near to impossible to get her up in the morning.
>
> **After:** Leona would sleep well and wake refreshed.

9

Fainting spells:
> **Before:** She would become weak to the point of fainting when she missed a meal.
>
> **After:** No incident of feeling faint or weak.

Personality:
> **Before:** Unreasonable rages, cranky, hard to handle.
>
> **After:** Pleasant, happy, loving, much better at communicating. She gets along better with siblings. No more door slamming.

Body temperature:
> **Before:** Always 97.6° F.
>
> **After:** Her body temperature rose to 98.6° F.

Ability to do household chores:
> **Before:** She could rarely finish a job. It was just too much. She put it off until later, or hunted for an excuse not to do them. Her bedroom was a disaster – cleaning it overwhelmed her. She only wanted to rest.
>
> **After:** She keeps her room reasonably clean and is able to do assigned tasks.

Physical appearance:
> **Before:** She was pale
>
> **After:** She is radiant and rosy-cheeked.

Feet:
> **Before:** Foul smelling.
>
> **After:** No unusual odor.

Skin:
> **Before:** Very sensitive; a scratch would leave a very red mark, especially in the neck area.
>
> **After:** Skin not sensitive.

General

Headaches, hives, and "growing pains" are also in the past. Leona is now able to tolerate some cigarette smoke.

Diary and Letters
November 20, 1994

Leona has not had a reaction after eating cheese. She is gradually losing her sensitivity to sugar and her school marks have improved dramatically.

There is no way we can ever thank Dr. Bateson-Koch for Leona's amazing return to the real world. Dr. Bateson-Koch is a true humanitarian. We shall be ever grateful for what she has done for our family.

August 7, 1995
Dear Dr. Bateson-Koch,

I am enclosing Leona's report card for 1993 - 1994 and 1994 - 1995. The first semester shows a lot of improvement but the last semester marks are even better. The 84.8% average is for both semesters. You can see the dramatic improvement from 68.3% in October 1993 when Leona was struggling to find out what was wrong with her - to the last term average of 87.7 in June of 1995 - a difference of 19.4% for the better!

May 11, 2001
Dear Dr. Bateson-Koch

We are still grateful to you for bringing Leona back to life. I consider my trip to see you as one of the best decisions in my life. What happened was nothing less than a miracle!!!

2

Allergy: The Multiple Symptom Syndrome

The greatest challenge with allergy is recognizing it. We have been conditioned to think of allergy in a limited capacity such as runny eyes, sniffling nose, sinus problems, skin rashes, asthma and hay fever. However, allergy is much more insidious and extensive. It can also take the form of arthritis, gall bladder disease, intractable headache, Crohn's disease, depression, psychotic behavior, and more than one hundred other conditions not normally thought of as allergy. Allergy does not cause every disease, but it can be involved in almost any disease and it can play an integral role in the development of disease. It is so prevalent that if you have not been told the cause of your health problems or symptoms, you should consider allergy first.

Allergy is not usually considered to be life threatening - who ever died from a runny nose? This lack of understanding persists in spite of the fact that almost everyone has heard about anaphylaxis, a massive allergic reaction that kills in minutes. Few other diseases can kill so rapidly. Anaphylaxis kills within sixteen minutes to two hours after contact with an allergen, whether it is from a bee sting, a handful of peanuts or a penicillin shot.

The slow progress of most allergies is even less understood. Over the course of months and years, allergy can so weaken the body systems that other life-threatening diseases gain a foothold in the body. This is because allergies, whether you recognize them or not, weaken the immune system over time so that the body cannot defend itself from foreign invaders and tissue degeneration. The most common way allergy kills is not by anaphylactic shock reaction, but by the slow, insidious, multiple-symptom syndrome.

How do you recognize allergy? You can suspect allergy any time you have an inflammation anywhere in your body. Allergy follows the cardinal signs of inflammation; pain, swelling, heat and redness. Whenever you have allergy, one and usually more of these symptoms are present. If the allergic reaction is near the skin, you will often see all four of these signs. For example, hives will produce the swelling, look red, feel warm, and be painful. Sometimes the reaction will occur internally where there are few nerve endings. In this case, the tissue may be swollen, red and hot, but you may not feel it because of the lack of nerve endings. Depending on where the reaction takes place, you will have different symptoms. Remember this little known fact: allergy can occur anywhere in the body, even in the brain. Inflammation is designated by words that end with itis. If an allergic reaction which produces inflammation occurs in the sinuses, it is called sinusitis; in the bowel, colitis; in the joints, arthritis; in the bronchi, bronchitis; and in the skin, dermatitis.

What Causes Allergy?

Allergy is the result of various insults to the body, coupled with a person's unique hereditary background and his or her individual metabolic state. Certain body patterns and metabolic states have been associated with the production of allergic symptoms. The fact that allergic disease is has many causes, has led to medical confusion; doctors look for only one cause, then try to find a drug to offset the symptoms. Since no single cause can be found, allergic symptoms are often ignored or attributed to mental or emotional stress.

Heredity

A person inherits the predisposition to allergy, rather than the specific allergy. Therefore it is the tendency to become allergic to a foreign substance, that is inherited. The greater the incidence of allergy in a family, the greater the tendency for the offspring to develop allergy. If one parent is allergic, the chances of the children being allergic are 50 to 58%. If both parents are allergic, the likelihood of the children being allergic is 67% to 100%.

Research confirms that a developing fetus in the uterus can demonstrate the hallmark of allergy, IgE antibody formation in the liver and lungs, by the eleventh week of gestation. IgE has also been found in the amniotic fluid (the fluid surrounding the fetus) at thirteen weeks. No IgE has been found in the arterial blood of the umbilical cord, leading doctors to believe that the placenta does not allow direct transfer of maternal blood containing IgE to the fetus. There are, however, studies that show that allergens transferred placentally can lead to intra-uterine sensitization. Allergies to penicillin, wheat, milk and eggs have been the most frequently documented.

Biochemical Individuality

A person's metabolic pattern or state is unique to that person. In some people the genetic requirements for nutrients can be much higher than normal to prevent disease. In others, metabolic individuality can cause them to react very differently to various substances.

Allergy appears to increase with advancing age. As a person ages, he tends to have weakened resistance due to a weakened immune system, various stages of organ degeneration, and having had more time to accumulate toxic substances which lead to metabolic overload. Also, nutritional deficiencies often increase as a person ages since they accumulate over time from the person's eating patterns.

Emotionally stressful situations can lead to diminished immune system function. Physical stress can increase nutrient requirements, leading to deficiency. Nutrient deficiency further stresses the immune system. Poor diet affects the body's ability to fight disease. It leaves the body unprotected. As one organ or body system loses its ability to function at peak performance, it affects other organs and systems. These other organs and systems must now do more work to compensate for the one that is stressed. As malnutrition continues, these accommodating organs and systems become stressed and lose their ability to function optimally. You cannot affect one part of the body without affecting other parts. According to James C. Breneman, MD, author of *Basics of Food Allergy*, food allergy and intolerance are technically, forms of malnutrition.

Toxic Load

Frequency and extent of exposure plays a large role in allergy. Increasing exposure to a substance causes toxic load to build faster in the body because it overburdens the body's detoxification pathways. Thousands of new chemicals are released into the environment every year, increasing exposure to a variety of industrial pollutants, pesticides and food additives. More than 6,000 new chemicals are tested in the United States each week. Over 7,000,000 distinct chemical compounds have appeared in scientific literature since 1965. All of these tend to work their way back into the human body. Today, the air, food and water have all been altered leading to varying degrees of toxic load.

Drugs

An average of 140,000 adverse drug reactions, causing death, occurs every year in the United States. Reactions to drugs have been well documented, although the information has not been well distributed. The drug most often causing allergic reactions is penicillin. The second most allergic drug is aspirin. Drugs contribute directly to allergy by decreasing liver function, increasing chemical overload and destroying enzyme systems.

Other drugs frequently associated with allergic reactions include:
Anti tuberculosis drugs
Antiarrhythmics (heart agents)
Anticonvulsant
Antimalarial drugs
Antipsychotic tranquilizers
Antiserum and vaccines
Blood pressure drugs
Heavy metals (including gold)
Sedative-hypnotics (barbiturates)
Sulfonamides

Infant Formula

Feeding infant formula to babies increases the frequency of allergy. Dr. Breneman states, "The highest incidence of lifetime milk allergy is found in this iatrogenically conditioned group." Iatrogenic means doctor-caused, presumably by prescribing cows milk infant formula.

Chronic Infections

Chronic, low-grade infections such as: bacterial, viral, fungal or parasitic, contribute heavily to the production of allergic symptoms. Long-standing infectious illness causes changes in the body that allow allergy to emerge. The body will react more readily to allergic stimuli because of damage to tissues and the extra work placed on the immune system. For example, asthma may occur after a bout with measles or pneumonia. Infection of the intestine can make its lining more permeable to undigested food particles, producing allergic symptoms. Biochemical changes take place in the body during prolonged illness, leading to decreased resistance to allergic stimuli. Toxins produced by the yeast Candida albicans play a major part in allergy. These toxins include acetaldehyde, carbon monoxide, alcohol, steroid substances and up to one hundred other substances not completely identified.

In general, the more frequent the exposure to a substance, the greater the incidence of allergy. Dr. Theron G. Randolph, a pioneer in clinical ecology, found that a person may acquire or lose sensitivities depending on how often they are exposed to a given food or substance. Dr. Randolph estimates that for every one allergy that we recognize, at least two more remain hidden.

Stress

Stress in any form, whether it is emotional, chemical, or environmental can contribute to allergic symptoms. Any stress that is beyond a person's ability to cope leads to adaptive changes physically and mentally. However, much mental stress has now been identified as being due to chemicals in the environment such as: Candida infections, toxins in food and electromagnetic disharmonies, previously unperceived by the individual.

Dental Fillings

Mercury is a component of the silver amalgam used in dental fillings. Mercury is highly toxic to the nerves and immune system. This toxicity has been historically documented as *mad hatter syndrome*, when hat makers became mentally ill after using mercury in the production of hats. Mercury in fillings of the teeth leeches out over the years. It also produces toxic mercury vapor in the mouth. Bacteria and fungi found in the mouth are capable of converting mercury into an even more toxic product called methyl mercury. Mercury is one of many toxins capable of contributing to chemical overload in the body, blocking enzymes and leading to degenerative diseases, including allergies.

Foods

Repeated consumption of a specific food plays a part in allergy by depleting enzyme systems. Most people eat only a very few foods, the ones they like best. For the majority of people, this is approximately fifteen foods, but they eat them in a variety of ways. If a person particularly likes potatoes, he will eat them frequently as baked potatoes, French fries, hash browns or potato chips. Beef may be steak, hamburger or stew. Daily overeating of a few specific foods has the effect of stressing the enzyme systems to handle that food. If the food is also an allergenic food, the body's capacity to deal with it is greatly diminished. Food is man's primary potential allergen and addictant. This is because everybody eats every day. As a result of the quantity eaten, food provides the greatest consistent stimulation to the body.

An article by Hugh A. Sampson, MD, which appeared in the *Journal of the American College of Nutrition* (Volume 9, Number 4, 1990), states, "The development of food allergy is the result of an interaction between food allergens, the gastrointestinal tract and the immune system."

Albert H. Rowe, MD, a pioneer on the subject of food allergy, has shown that food allergy can be responsible for any symptom in any system of the body and it can manifest itself at any age.

Airborne Inhalants

In some people, pollens, dust spores, insect debris, animal dander, and airborne chemicals play a major role in allergy, by stimulating allergic reactions to take place, and creating toxic overload of the immune system. When these people also use tobacco, alcohol and drugs, the body can be stressed even more and at an earlier age.

Understanding Allergy

The word allergic implies that the allergenic substance is the cause. In fact, this only demonstrates that the person, for one reason or another, has lost the normal ability to cope appropriately with that substance. The substance itself is not the cause; it is only the trigger of the allergic reaction.

Many allergic symptoms are characteristically ignored. No one disputes that classic symptoms such as runny nose, watery eyes and skin rashes are allergic conditions. No one disputes that allergy is involved when a person bites into a peanut butter cookie and dies of anaphylactic shock. It is amazing that if allergy can produce symptoms as mild as a runny nose or as life threatening as anaphylactic shock, that the range of symptoms between these two extremes is seldom recognized. Why are these intermediary symptoms rarely linked to allergy?

For the most part, professionals have not been taught to recognize these symptoms as being of allergic origin. Although new information is becoming available, it is still too often tucked away on the shelves of medical libraries rather than being used.

Any symptom which your body is capable of producing can be of allergic origin. Not every symptom is allergy, but any symptom can be allergy. What about ulcers, high blood pressure, gall bladder disease, bed-wetting, and arthritis or enlarged prostate? New information is showing that these conditions can be of allergic origin. We now have volumes of reports from all over the world indicating that allergy can involve any part of the body.

The field of allergy is evolving although there is still much controversy among professionals as to causes of allergy, appropriate testing, terminology, and definitions of allergy and other altered reactions. To understand these differences, it is helpful to look into the background of allergy.

3

Dogma Limits Healing

Allergy is not new. The symptoms of allergy have been described since ancient times. The death in 2641 B.C. of King Menes, an Egyptian pharaoh, after being stung by a bee, sounds very much like what we describe as anaphylactic shock. The Babylonian Talmud offered advice on building up tolerance to eggs in persons who experienced distress after eating them. About 99 B.C., Lucretius said," What is food to one man may be fierce poison to others."

Around 1906, things started to change. The term allergy was coined from two Greek words meaning altered reactivity. It meant that an allergy was an adverse response to a substance by one person but not by most people. For example, pollen could give some people symptoms such as runny nose and eyes, but others experienced no reaction. At about the same time, Frances Hare, an Australian physician, wrote two volumes titled, *The Food Factor in Disease*. These volumes detailed cases in which many common symptoms including mental symptoms are linked to eating common foods.

For the next twenty years doctors documented reactions to specific food allergens. However, the vast array of symptoms, coupled with the vast array of causative agents, including food, chemicals and inhalants, presented problems from a scientific standpoint. How do you study a substance that seemingly causes headaches in one person, rashes in another and depression in yet another, particularly when the same substance causes no demonstrable symptoms in most people?

In 1926, a milestone decision was made. European allergists met with American allergists and agreed to limit the definition of allergy to immunological types of reactions only. Reactions involving the

21

immune system produce antibodies in the tissues. Here was physical evidence that could be categorized and measured. Before 1926, allergy was considered to be any altered reaction to a common substance. After 1926, allergies were allergen-antibody reactions involving the immune system only. This decision was reinforced around 1967 when the immunoglobulin IgE was discovered. IgE was the first recognized antibody involved in immune-type reactions and became the classic marker for allergy. This historic decision severely limited the scope of allergy for the next 50 years.

Following the 1926 decision, two groups of allergists appeared. The scientific, orthodox allergists, who worked primarily with molds, dusts, grasses and pollens, required an allergen-antibody reaction as a basis for diagnosis. The other group was considered unorthodox, as it persisted studying foods and other substances, even though an immunological reaction could not necessarily be found. Research grants from major food manufacturers went mostly to the orthodox groups, which reinforced the narrow definition of allergy.

Even today, traditional allergists tend to diagnose only reactions involving IgE antibody production as being allergy. Any other reactions and symptoms are likely to be ignored. *The Atlas of Allergies* by Philip Fireman, MD and Raymond G. Slavin, MD states, "This immunologic definition of allergy is accepted by almost all, but not every allergist since non-immune processes can influence the pathogenesis of allergic diseases with recognized immune etiologies."

Food sensitivities often do not produce immunological reactions from skin testing, although they may produce a wide variety of symptoms throughout the body. Therefore, they may not be considered to be allergies. Many doctors now estimate that up to two-thirds of allergic-like reactions may be in this category.

In 1965, Dr. Randolph Moss, along with other doctors, founded the Society for Clinical Ecology. These doctors recognized the ecological aspects, including the effects of foods, in many medical problems. Unfortunately, clinical ecology is not taught in medical schools. Doctors learn about it through postgraduate courses, private reading and clinical observations.

Terminology; Controversy Causes Confusion

Many terms have evolved over the years to describe both allergic and various other adverse reactions. Examples include the following: hypersensitivity, intolerance, idiosyncrasy, maladaptive, allergic-like, atopic, and sensitivity. For a word that is less than 100 years old, allergy has been defined, redefined and disputed more than its share. Fortunately, in the last few years, there is a coming together on this issue. While there are still those physicians who disagree, a broader definition of allergy is becoming more accepted. Although the classic allergic reaction is still considered a reaction with an IgE antibody, other forms of adverse reactions are being identified and recognized, and more and more doctors have come full circle and are accepting the use of the word allergy to mean simply altered reactivity. An allergen is any substance that is capable of initiating an allergic reaction. It is recognized by the body as foreign and induces an immune response with the production of antibodies.

An antibody is any of the immunoglobulins (IgE, IgG, IgA, IgM) that are produced in response to a specific allergen and that counteracts the effect of that allergen.

Agreement has been harder to reach when it comes to the definition of adverse food reactions but fortunately, in the last ten years, more agreement has emerged on the following terms:

Food Allergy

Food allergy is usually any adverse reaction to food in which the immune system is demonstrably involved. This must usually be demonstrated through laboratory testing and characteristically involves a reaction where the IgE antibody is identified. This is considered a true food allergy.

Food Intolerance

Food intolerance is any other adverse reaction to food in which the involvement of the immune system is unproven. However, these adverse reactions can often produce symptoms clinically indistinguishable from food allergy. Further, although immune involvement cannot be deciphered, this does not exclude the possibility that the immune system may be involved. Food intolerance may occur from the food itself, from additives or chemicals that are in the food, from naturally occurring toxins in the food or even from metabolic disorders of the person involved.

Food Sensitivity

Food sensitivity is a common catchall term employed for food allergy, food intolerance and other adverse reactions to food. Proof of food allergy is still often difficult to establish. Most laboratory blood tests deal primarily in identifying the IgE antibody and often do not screen for reactions that may produce the IgG, IgA or IgM antibodies. It is interesting to note that the most accepted diagnostic test for allergy, the elimination diet and subsequent reintroduction of suspected substances, does not differentiate between the two terms, allergy and intolerance.

The Vital Choice: Relief or Wellness?
Antihistamines

There are many medicinal products on the market that promise to relieve, control, manage or attack allergy. These products work by interfering with various chemical reactions that normally occur in the body. An example is antihistamines. These drugs may relieve symptoms by preventing histamine from being released from certain cells in the body.

While antihistamines are the most common drugs used to treat allergic symptoms, they are not without side effects. A major side effect is drowsiness. Driving a motor vehicle or operating machinery is not recommended while under the influence of antihistamines. Another common side effect is dryness of the mouth, nose and throat. Blurred vision, dizziness, loss of appetite, nausea, upset stomach, low blood pressure, headache and loss of co-ordination are less common side effects. Antihistamines sometimes cause nervousness, restlessness or insomnia.

Amphetamine-like Products

Many over-the-counter products sold for allergies contain amphetamine-like nasal decongestants. Adverse reactions to these products include jitteriness, sleeplessness and potential heart problems. At any rate, relief or control of symptoms is all that is offered. There is a difference between relieving or controlling a symptom and actually getting well. Using drugs to manage and control allergy does not get you well. However, people have become well by using alternative, natural methods which do not attack allergy, but instead promote the body's natural healing response and help to remove conditions in the body which are stressing the body's immune system.

By understanding more about allergy and by stimulating the body's healing response, it is possible to recover from allergies without having to get rid of the family pet, without moving from your home, without allergy shots, without rotating foods and keeping diet diaries and without cooking allergy-free recipes for the rest of your life.

Dr. William Philpott states,

We must always keep in mind that the greatest enemy of any science, or any discovery of truth, is a closed mind. Accordingly, we should continue to seek the courage to ask impertinent questions which will shake out complacency and challenge our minds to look deeper into the great mystery of the human body.

4

Five Key Concepts about Allergy

The new, broader understanding of allergy is based on five essential concepts.

Five Key Concepts about Allergy

Concept One: Balance: The Essence of Health

Concept Two: Any Symptom Can Be Allergy

Concept Three: Symptoms Appear when Allergic Load is Reached

Concept Four: Allergy Has No Single Cause

Concept Five: Self-Empowerment through Personal Responsibility

Concept One:
Balance: The Essence of Health

Your body is incredibly dynamic. Millions of activities take place in your body each second, mostly without your awareness. For example, seven to ten million new cells are formed every second. All of the blood in the circulatory system flows through your body an average of once a minute when your body is at rest. It circulates about six times a minute during exercise.

At the same time, the blood is carrying oxygen and nutrients to all of the estimated 70 to 100 trillion cells in your body. It is estimated that one food molecule requires up to 10 million 2-way electrical transmissions to go from the original food to the cell. The body's capacity is so great that if you were able to take all the DNA out of the cells and stretch it into a single line, calculations indicate that it would circle the earth 5 million times.

Your body has the wisdom to take care of all its structures and activities and to heal itself without your conscious help. In a healthy body all of the organs and tissues perform functions that help maintain conditions of equilibrium (homeostasis).

As long as nothing intervenes, the body will remain running perfectly. If trauma or other irritation occurs to the body, it will make the necessary corrections through compensation to return to a state of balance. Even if the traumatic irritation is prolonged, the body will still strive to make corrections by calling in other systems or substituting other materials to stay balanced. However, if the stress becomes overwhelming, eventually some of these compensating systems may become exhausted. The body then cannot return to homeostasis and remains out of balance. This is like a gyroscope starting to wind down: it simply cannot run smoothly and efficiently anymore and starts to wobble. Visible symptoms then develop.

The primary sources of prolonged trauma and irritation to the body are habits, lifestyle and beliefs. For example, drinking alcohol every day is a source of irritation for the body. The body tries to compensate for the loss of minerals, the lack of oxygen and the toxicity to the liver. If the stress continues long enough, the body will go out of balance and call in compensatory mechanisms in order to survive. Regular over-consumption of alcohol is an example of a habit affecting homeostasis.

For every action in the body, there is also an opposite action. You have muscles to open your hand and other muscles to close your hand. You have hormones to speed up metabolism and hormones to slow it down. The body stays in balance by constantly making adjustments day and night, day after day and year after year. It's sort of like staying in the middle of a teeter-totter. Then along comes a lifestyle that pushes you out to one end. Eventually, the exhausted body cannot make its way back to the middle. Symptoms appear. The body is telling you that it is not in homeostasis and a correction should be made allowing the body to move back toward health. If this is not done, that symptom will eventually turn into something more serious.

Eczema in the infant often becomes asthma in the adult. Low blood sugar often becomes adult onset diabetes. When an allergic symptom appears, the body is saying that it is struggling to cope with its environment, both internal and external. It is imperative to change something now to take stress off the body. A body that is in homeostasis cannot be exhibiting allergy. It will not react abnormally to any substance. A body in balance does not have any symptoms. It has only health.

Concept Two:
Any Symptom Can Be Allergy.

Any symptom or condition of the body, anywhere in the body, at any time, can be allergy, particularly when that symptom is not explainable in other terms. Food allergies in particular are poorly understood. When you eat a banana and get an immediate pain in your abdomen or stomach, you realize that there is a connection between eating the banana and getting the pain. But if the only response to that banana comes days later in the form of a swollen joint, you do not necessarily recognize that there is a relationship between what you ate and the response that occurred. Much masked or delayed allergy falls into this category.

Allergy is considered an altered reaction – the reaction that one person will get to a substance that does not affect other people. Anything a person puts in his or her mouth is capable of eliciting an allergic response, even tap water. It's not the water itself but what is in the water, such as chlorine, fluoride and up to one hundred other chemicals, that can precipitate the reaction. A person can also have an allergic response to the air that he or she breathes. This is, of course, more readily understood, because we have a greater awareness of the toxicity of tobacco smoke and city smog and the effects of pollen.

Doctors who have worked extensively with allergy, and especially with food allergy, are astounded at the wide range of symptoms that can be observed in patients. It is an extraordinary concept that PMS, epilepsy, bloody diarrhea, backache and swollen arthritic joints can be produced by common everyday foods. The idea that foods, considered nourishment for the body, are capable of producing a major illness may be difficult to comprehend.

Milk is the most common allergen. The patient who drinks lots of milk is aghast when it turns out to be a cause of his or her colitis. This patient may have believed that he was doing something good for himself. A person who drinks gallons of milk often turns out to be calcium deficient. How can this possibly be, he wonders? If you react allergically to a food, it is difficult for the body to absorb its nutrients.

Dr. James C. Breneman writes, "The incidence of diet-related problems is greater than the incidence of any other type of illness affecting mankind." He estimates that 60% of the population has unknown food allergies or intolerance's. Other authors estimate the figure to be closer to 80%. It is important that people increase their awareness of the scope of allergy as a possible cause of their symptoms. Most people do not think of gall bladder symptoms as being caused by allergy, especially if they have never had classic allergic symptoms such as hay fever or skin rashes. Many people have little awareness that bed-wetting in a child can be allergy, especially to milk. This is particularly true when the child does not appear to have any other allergic symptoms. One patient, after reciting a long list of symptoms, remarked that she did not have any allergies; all she had was arthritis. She did not realize that allergy often plays a role in this disease. If you have allergic symptoms that are not the traditional type, you will often be told there is nothing wrong with you, or that it is, all in your mind.

Doctors have limited awareness and knowledge of food allergy because of the following reasons:

1. Food allergy is not taught at medical schools.
2. Doctors must get training in food allergy from post-graduate seminars or from clinical experience.
3. Many doctors consider food allergy to be fantasy.
4. Orthodox allergists recognize only immunological-type reactions. They do not consider anything else to be allergy, even in the face of obvious clinical symptoms.

If the scope of allergy has not been taught to doctors, how are they to recognize it? The fact is that most allergy goes untreated and unrecognized while the patient must put up with chronic debilitating symptoms.

Concept Three:
Symptoms Appear when Allergic Load is Reached.
Allergic load is the amount of chemicals, food allergens and

inhalant pollutants that a person can be exposed to before symptoms appear. It is the sum total of toxicity (toxic load) accumulated before systems in the body malfunction, produce symptoms and alert you to the fact that something is wrong.

In the book *Clinical Ecology*, Dr. Lawrence Dickey writes,

It would be surprising if people were not allergic to pesticides put into the ground and sprayed on crops, to flour improvers, anti-staling agents, emulsifying compounds, artificial colorings, preservatives and the whole terrifying array of potentially toxic substances now being added to our food in order to improve appearance, flavor, shelf-life and profitability.

It is estimated that 8 to 15 pounds of these toxic materials are taken into each person's body each year. The combined and accumulated effects are not known, but we are seeing an increase of observable abnormal reactions in the body. Because the immune system is programmed to defend us from foreign substances, allergy or intolerance is one of the body's initial responses. After many years of being in a hyper-excited state, the immune system becomes exhausted. This leaves the body with lowered defenses, which can later lead to many forms of chronic degenerative disease.

It is not known whether the human body has built sufficient enzyme systems to eliminate or neutralize all the toxic effects of the smorgasbord of chemicals taken in. It is known that oxidative enzymes and certain vitamins and minerals are necessary to eliminate or neutralize the toxins. However, with pounds of chemicals going into the body each year, year after year, the question remains – are we are over-taxing our body's ability to produce the substances necessary to eliminate the chemicals? As the nutrient value of our food goes down and the chemical content rises, can our bodies meet the demand? When the demand is greater than the supply, the body must pull in compensatory mechanisms in order to defend itself.

Allergic or toxic load is different for everyone. People are born with varying genetic strengths and weaknesses. The child of an alcoholic mother has a much smaller health reserve to start with than the child of a healthy mother. Toxic load also depends upon what you are exposed to. Before it was known how toxic asbestos is, workers in asbestos factories built up toxic load of asbestos in their lungs faster than people of the general population. When a point of toxicity is reached in the body from any source, whether it is ingested, inhaled, injected or absorbed through the skin, allergy is one of the first symptoms to appear. That swollen joint, headache or gastritis is a sign telling you something is wrong. If you ignore these signs, you can expect increasingly severe symptoms.

In the book *The McDougall Plan*, Dr. John A. McDougall states, The body's immune system has a limited capacity to deal with allergens and when the system becomes overloaded, allergic symptoms appear. If you can reduce the intake of allergens from one source, such as food, you will ease the burden on the entire immune system. In this way you can help your body deal with other sources of allergies, such as particles in the air.

Each person's ability to metabolize toxins, pollens, foods and chemicals can differ considerably according to his or her own biochemical makeup. Almost every food available in a modern supermarket has been tampered with in some way, to the detriment of its nutritional and enzyme content. Unless it is certified organically grown, all fresh produce has been sprayed, has been grown on mineral-deficient soil and has absorbed constituents of artificial fertilizers, which may contain herbicides.

Some produce has been irradiated, which destroys its enzyme content. Boxed foods are all enzyme-deficient, as they are processed at high temperatures, and they may also contain chemical additives. Frozen foods may be blanched or cooked and often contain salt, sugar and chemical additives. Canned foods are subjected to very high temperatures, destroying their enzymes and some nutrients. All this contributes toward the individual's toxic load, regardless of his or her resistance level.

Concept Four:
Allergy Has No Single Cause.

For many diseases, there is no such thing as a cause. We are told through the media that scientists are looking for the cause of cancer and the cause of arthritis. Why is it assumed that there is only one cause? The truth is that in chronic conditions, there isn't. That there is only one cause for each disease is an assumption that will eventually be proven wrong for many degenerative conditions.

The problem is that the one-cause-one-disease model is the only one that fits current scientific testing criteria. Robert C. Atkins, MD, in his book *Dr. Atkins' Health Revolution,* explains that the double blind study is the criterion scientists use:

> The double blind is an excellent test for evaluating pharmaceutical and single variables. I agree with that; when it is applicable, it should be used. The problem is that, as the protocols get stricter in their exclusion of subjectivity, the area of applicability becomes narrower and narrower. The real blind spot in the double blind is that the leadership in medicine continues to insist upon it as the only acceptable proof, even though its applicability is so limited. The problem is that for many good therapies, a double-blind protocol cannot even be devised.

A good example of this problem is provided by nutrients such as vitamins or minerals, which are never found alone in nature. A nutrient may not test well as a single entity because it needs synergistic nutrients which work together to enhance its action. As a single nutrient, a vitamin may produce a weak effect. For example, vitamin C as ascorbic acid (a single nutrient) may be required in higher doses, but when used in conjunction with bioflavonoids will produce a better result with a lower dose.

Allergy is the cumulative effect of many insults to the body which, over time, have overwhelmed the body's protective mechanisms. While dust may appear to be the cause of your runny nose, in reality it is only the trigger that activates the symptoms in an already compromised organism.

Concept Five:
Self-Empowerment through Personal Responsibility
True healing is movement toward health, balance, and wholeness. Healing also involves the acceptance of responsibility for one's health. Healing takes place on many levels and in many different ways but the one constant is that healing always involves a change. A basic

tenet of healing is that the most effective way for an afflicted person to improve his or her health is to seek out new information, approaches, and ideas and to apply them.

Continuing to do the same things in the same way will reinforce keeping the same health problems because many of those usual, comfortable habits are often what created the ill health in the first place. Although change may seem difficult or uncomfortable, it can also be fun and exciting.

Medical studies show that when a person has control, or plays a part in his or her own recovery, that there is a better outcome. Therefore, becoming an active participant in your own health care, discovering the causes of your health challenges and dealing with them yourself leads to many rewards; the pride of accomplishment, a healthy, more energetic body, and personal empowerment.

Health is your responsibility. Remember the old saying – you can lead a horse to water but you can't make him drink ? It's the same with health. You can be shown the path to better health, but only you can follow the path. You can learn what foods to eat, but only you can choose whether or not to eat them

Because the body is self-healing, the power to be healthy is within you at this very moment. All you need to do is discover how to tap into that power to obtain health. It is up to you to learn what it is that your body needs. Your medical doctor looks only for disease and medical tests are designed to either diagnose or eliminate the possibility of disease. Tests are not done to determine your individual biochemical requirements to stay healthy. Your body will stay healthy as long as you give it what it needs and do not negatively interfere with it, either knowingly or unknowingly. That could mean changing your lifestyle, diet or beliefs. It is your responsibility to make those changes if you wish to be healthy. Disease, including allergy, is the result of a lifetime of destructive habits. If you don't like the result, you must change the input.

Health is a choice. Anyone desiring to be healthy can decide to make the changes necessary to accomplish that goal. Taking personal responsibility leads to wellness.

5

The Fascinating Life of an Allergen

The immune system is the primary defense system. It is located throughout the body and comprised of a master gland called the thymus plus the spleen, tonsils, lymph nodes, adrenals, appendix, bone marrow, specialized lymphoid tissue, white blood cells (lymphocytes), mast cells, antibodies, complement proteins and many chemical mediators. Lymphocytes are major defenders of the body and billions of these tiny cells patrol the blood stream looking for and destroying invading viruses, bacteria, parasites and other foreign substances.

Normal body cells are coated with a special protective protein that the immune system can recognize. Because of this protective coat, normal cells are not attacked by the immune system. Dead tissues and foreign particles have no protective coat, and are phagocytized (eaten) by cells of the immune system.

A person can become sensitized when a foreign substance enters the body by any means. It could happen by inhalation, ingestion, injection or absorption through the skin. When a person is exposed to this foreign substance, antibodies are built by plasma cells of the immune system. When the substance or allergen is taken in again, it reacts with the specified antibodies. As the allergen contacts an antibody, an immediate reaction takes place, producing symptoms, usually within minutes or hours.

However, when an allergen reacts with lymphocytes, a delayed form of allergy may occur This delayed form, occurring hours or even days later is not nearly so well recognized by professionals. For example, if you eat strawberries and hives appear within hours, you will probably realize that strawberries were a precipitating factor. But if the symptoms appear two to three days later you often will have forgotten by then that you ate strawberries and you are less likely to link the two events together.

Allergic reaction runs one of two courses: symptoms can appear and subsequently disappear, or they can produce permanent pathological changes. Understanding how these reactions occur, and how they affect the tissues of the body, gives us clues not only on how to recognize them but also to eliminate them.

The Classic (IgE) Allergic Reaction

Classic cases of allergic reaction involve antibodies, which are gamma globulins called *immunoglobulins*. IgE antibodies are synthesized by plasma cells located primarily under the mucosal surfaces of the respiratory and digestive tract. Antibodies make up about 20% of the plasma proteins of the body. There are five major types: IgE, IgG, IgM, IgA and IgD. 75% of the antibodies in a normal person are of the IgG type. IgE makes up only a small proportion, about 1%, but it is particularly involved in allergy. It is the IgE antibody that the allergist looks for when diagnosing allergy. After the IgE antibody is formed, it becomes bound to receptor sites on white blood cells known as mast cells and basophils. A single blood basophil can have up to 100,000 IgE receptor sites. A non-allergic person will have only 20 to 50% of the receptors bound by antibodies. But nearly 100% of the sites will be occupied by IgE in an allergic individual.

Once IgE is bound to these sites the cells are considered to be sensitized. When the specific allergen is introduced again, a cascade of biochemical reactions takes place. This is the classic allergic reaction. The mast cells and basophils release potent chemicals into the tissues. The tissues most commonly affected are the smooth muscles of blood vessels, bronchioles and collagen or connective tissues. However, any tissue of the body can be affected. Antibodies can be formed in the blood stream and circulate. They attach to cells at other sites in the body. When re-exposed to the specific allergen, the allergic reaction takes place in what is now known as the "shock tissue."

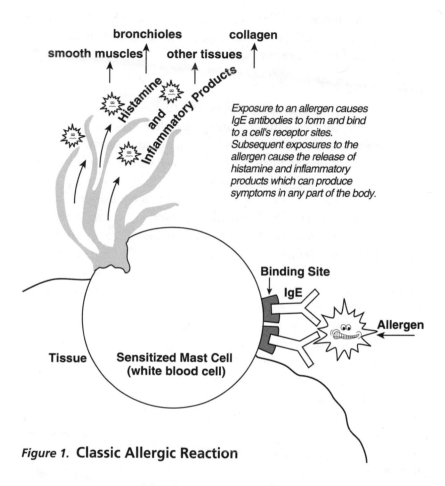

Figure 1. **Classic Allergic Reaction**

IgG

IgG immunoglobulins make up three-fourths of the antibodies of the blood stream. They are produced by white blood cells known as B-lymphocytes. IgG can attack and destroy most bacteria. Some researchers believe that IgG is involved in up to two-thirds of all allergic reactions. IgG plays an important role in activating the complement system. Complement is a collective term used to describe about twenty different proteins, many of which are enzyme precursors. When IgG attaches to an invader or allergen, the comple-

37

ment system moves in. Through a series of chemical reactions in which the cell wall of the invader is eaten by the complement system enzymes, the invader ruptures and dies.

IgA

It has been more recently discovered that the immunoglobulin IgA plays a major role in protection against allergy. Secretory IgA antibodies are found in saliva, tears, the blood stream and especially along the lining of the digestive tract. IgA's major role is to defend against foreign substances before they can enter the body.

Since the digestive system is often the first to contact an allergen, this is the place where significant allergic reactions occur. If an allergen is able to get past the IgA and enter the blood stream, it can be an indication of a deficiency of the secretory IgA that lines the digestive tract. This is why IgA can be considered a front line defender against allergens. Secretory IgA binds the allergens so that these compounds can be neutralized.

Statistics indicate that almost one-half of Americans are lacking secretory IgA. This means that allergens can penetrate the intestinal membranes unopposed and reach the blood stream. In addition, when an allergic food is eaten, some amount of secretory IgA is used up. If allergic food is eaten on a regular basis, this can contribute to secretory IgA deficiency.

In non-allergenic people, 3,000 to 5,000 milligrams of secretory IgA are produced daily. Allergic persons secrete substantially less secretory IgA than normal, and some persons secrete close to none at all.

Some Drugs which can Contribute to Secretory IgA Deficiency

Antacids	Birth control pill	Indocin
Antibiotics	Clinoril	Naprosyn
Aspirin	Cortisone	Tagamet

Products of Allergic Reactions

Several substances are released in allergic reactions, causing far-reaching effects on tissue. These substances are described below.

Histamine

Histamine is a natural substance liberally distributed throughout the body, especially in the skin, heart, lungs, gastrointestinal mucosa and brain. It is the best known of the inflammatory substances released by mast cells of the tissues during an adverse reaction. It quickly spreads into the surrounding tissue. Histamine acts directly on the small blood vessels making them leaky to the fluid of the body. This in turn leads to edema (swelling of the tissue), which then acts on nerve endings, causing pain.

When histamine is released three major reactions result.

1. Smooth muscles contract. If this occurs in the bronchi, this reduces the diameter of the airways, which means less air enters the lungs.
2. Vasodilation increases blood flow to the tissues, which then become red, warm, and swollen.
3. Vascular permeability increases, which allows material inside of the blood vessels to leak into the surrounding tissue.

Common Symptoms of Histamine

Anxiety and agitation sometimes with odd body sensations

Fast heartbeat, palpitations, irregular beats

Headache

Increased acid secretion to the stomach causing pain and/or small intestine contracts, causing cramps

Itching, burning, flushing skin

Local nose swelling, congestion, sneezing, or asthma

Foods containing high amounts of histamines include fish, shellfish, tomatoes, pork, venison, and eggs.

Kinins

Few doctors recognize kinin reactions as a source of intense pain. Kinins are a group of chemicals released into tissues as a result of inflammation. Of these, bradykinin is the most important. Bradykinin is one of the most potent vasodilators (dilators of blood vessels) known. It is about ten times more active than histamine or serotonin. It may be involved in up to two-thirds of allergic reactions.

Bradykinin causes intense pain, as it is a very powerful stimulator of pain receptors. It also contracts smooth muscle, increases vascular permeability and dilates peripheral arterioles.

Leukotrienes

Leukotrienes are potent inflammatory substances that were first identified in 1979. Leukotrienes play an especially important role in asthma since they are highly inflammatory and can cause smooth muscle contraction. They are produced or secreted by various immune cells such as: mast cells, macrophages, eosinophils, basophils and monocytes. Leukotrienes produce powerful bronchoconstriction, accumulation of mucus, and swelling in the respiratory tissue. It is estimated that leukotrienes are 1000 times more inflammatory than histamine. Leukotrienes stimulate the production of other inflammatory substances such as platelet activating factor and some of the prostaglandins.

Other Substances

Other powerful substances that play a role in allergic disorders are prostaglandins and thromboxanes. Prostaglandins are chemical substances that have been identified more recently. When activated, these hormones can cause powerful inflammation. Prostaglandins exist in almost every tissue of the body. They can have both vasoconstricting and vasodilating effects.

Common Thread

What do all these substances have in common? They are all vasoactive, causing blood vessels to dilate or contract, and they are all inflammatory, causing swelling, heat and pain. The dilation of local blood vessels causes loss of fluid into the tissue. Along with this fluid comes increased numbers of proteins. The proteins tend to cluster in the tissues. These clusters are difficult for the lymphatics to absorb, so the proteins tend to pool there. The proteins pull water out of the circulation, causing swelling. These clustered proteins attract excess sodium, which attracts still more fluid. Excess fluid and excess sodium create a lack of oxygen supply to the cells. This causes even more cell injury because cells need oxygen to survive. Decreased oxygen slows down cell function and causes acid to accumulate in the cell. It is believed that ischemic (lacking in blood) tissues also release toxins such as histamine, serotonin and tissue enzymes. Eventually the cells die.

Immune Complexes

A common consequence of allergic reaction is the binding together of allergens and antibodies to form large allergen-antibody (immune) complexes. When formed, these immune complexes are deposited in tissues such as the kidneys, lungs, small blood vessels, liver and uterus. They can also be deposited in the arteries of the brain (e.g. migraine sufferers) and in the brain membranes. Immune complexes release substances that activate a cascade of biochemical reactions. Additionally, complexes are capable of at least temporarily clogging up joints and blood vessels, resulting in local tissue injury. They can damage the filtering organs of the body, such as the kidneys and lymphatics. Immune complexes are responsible for up to 90% of kidney disease in humans. An increase in the permeability of the small blood vessels is required for these large immune complexes to be deposited in the various tissues. Histamine paves the way by causing leaking of the capillaries.

Anaphylaxis

The most life-threatening and dramatic of all allergic reactions is anaphylaxis. It occurs so rapidly that often therapy cannot be applied before death occurs. Anaphylaxis involves the whole body, causing similar shock symptoms to those one might see in a car accident victim. Symptoms begin within minutes of exposure to the allergen. Since the symptoms involve the whole body, the reaction is immediate and explosive. The victim may experience in rapid succession...a constricted feeling in the chest, dizziness, wheezing, nausea, vomiting or diarrhea, weakness, hoarseness, abdominal pain, skin manifestations, swelling and cyanosis (turning blue). Blood pressure can fall rapidly, and unconsciousness and death follows.

The number one cause of anaphylaxis is drugs, especially injected drugs. Injecting a substance bypasses the normal defense system of the body. Penicillin is the most common drug involved in anaphylaxis, with aspirin running a close second. Dyes used in X-ray diagnosis have also caused anaphylaxis, as have some anesthetics used in surgery. Peanuts and other nuts, eggs, fish and shellfish are the most common foods involved in anaphylaxis. Sulfites added to fruits, vegetables and processed foods are another frequent cause. Less common, but every bit as important, are the stinging insects. Every year, bees and wasps cause anaphylaxis.

Chronic Immune Suppression

Allergic reactions have a boomerang effect on the immune system. Although the immune system initially responds with a heightened reaction when an allergen is contacted, the white blood cell population then becomes depressed and remains lower than normal for as long as the exposure continues. This can cause chronic suppression of the immune system if the allergen is consumed or contacted on a daily basis.

6

Evidence of Allergy

Allergies to foods and environmental substances produce symptoms that go far beyond the familiar sneeze, wheeze, scratch and itch generally associated with allergies. They can be responsible for a wide array of symptoms. Dr. Albert Rowe, an early pioneer on this subject, published a book in 1931, which demonstrated how food allergy was responsible for a wide range of symptoms, which can affect any part of the body and can begin at any age.

It is important to note that allergens do not necessarily cause their major symptoms at the place where they first come into contact with the body. They may enter by one route and then cause symptoms somewhere else in the body because they are carried to that point by the blood. For example, inhaled allergens may cause skin reactions because they enter the bloodstream through the membranes of the nose or lung and are then circulated by the blood to the skin. Food allergy can trigger the bronchoconstriction that we see in asthma. In addition, it is increasingly apparent that when allergy affects the central nervous system (brain and spinal cord), the result can be mood swings ranging from depression to manic-depressive and psychotic disorders and all the symptoms in between.

To date, over one hundred symptoms have been recognized as being caused by allergic reactions to foods and environmental chemicals. No part of the body is immune to allergy.

Allergic Reactions to Foods and Environmental Chemicals – Most Common Medically recognized Symptoms.

Neurological Symptoms

Amnesia

Apathy

Aphasia (inability to speak)

Blackouts

Coma

Delusions

Depression

Disorientation

Dizziness

Emotional instability

Epilepsy

Fainting

Fatigue

Feeling of indecision

Hallucinations

Headache

Hyperactivity

Impaired comprehension

Impaired coordination

Irritability

Lethargy

Melancholy (sad feelings)

Mental lapses

Moodiness

Nervousness

Neuralgia

Paranoid thinking

Sleeplessness (insomnia)

Stammering

Violent behavior

Withdrawal

Joint Symptoms

Arthralgia (joint pain)

Arthritis

Swollen ankles

Circulatory Symptoms

Anemia

Angina pectoris (heart pain)

Chest pain

Edema

Hypertension (High blood pressure)

Irregular heartbeat

Irregular pulse

Phlebitis

Respiratory Symptoms

Asthma

Bronchitis

Coughing

Runny nose

Sinusitis

Wheezing, shortness of breath

Gastrointestinal Symptoms

Abdominal pain

Belching

Bloating

Canker sores

Colitis

Constipation

Diarrhea

Diverticulitis

Duodenal ulcer

Excessive gas

Food cravings

Gagging

Gall bladder pain

Heartburn

Hemorrhoids

Hunger pains

Indigestion

Nausea

Peptic ulcers

Salivation

Stomach cramps

Vomiting

Skin Symptoms

Acne

Bleeding and bruising

Clammy skin

Eczema

Hives

Itching

Sweating

Tendency towards cracked skin

Muscle-skeletal Symptoms

Backache

Myalgia (muscle pain)

Neck ache

Hormonal Symptoms

Dysmenorrhea

Frigidity

Impotence

Other Symptoms

Bed-wetting

Cataracts

Conjunctivitis

Diabetes

Failure to thrive (in infants)

Fever

Hoarseness

Lower blood sugar

Multiple sclerosis

Obesity

Otitis media

(inflammation, discharge

  from ear, earaches)

  Sneezing spells

Swelling around the eyes

Tinnitus (ringing of the ear)

The Gastrointestinal Tract

More symptoms of food allergy arise in the tissue of the gastrointestinal tract than in any other tissue of the body. Foods have direct contact for the longest time with the lining of the digestive tract, which can establish sensitization. This is especially true for the stomach, the duodenum (small intestine) and the rectum. Antibodies coat the mucosa (lining) of the gastrointestinal tract to act as a barrier to the external world.

When an allergic reaction occurs here, the released products such as histamine cause inflammation in the mucosa, which becomes more permeable. Large particles (macromolecules) of incompletely digested food can then be absorbed through the mucosa and gain entrance to the blood stream. Once in the blood stream, these particles can be carried to any part of the body. Studies have shown that when the stomach has an absent or diminished supply of hydrochloric acid, even more macromolecules are found to be absorbed by the intestine, due to the fact that there are more particles present. Also, when trypsin, a pancreatic protein-digesting enzyme, is inhibited, more macromolecules are absorbed. Another study showed that low stomach acid results in increased formation of antibodies to cow's milk. The body reacts to macromolecules in the blood stream by producing more antibodies. Other ways the intestinal lining can become damaged are prolonged bacterial, viral, or yeast infection, parasites, toxins, decreased oxygen supply to the mucosa and X-radiation used in treating cancer.

Digestive diseases are the second highest cause of doctor visits. Common intestinal conditions associated with food allergy include: ulcers, sores in the mouth, colic, diarrhea, constipation, hemorrhoids, colitis and Crohn's disease.

The Stomach

Allergic reactions that occur in the stomach lead to the release of histamine from the mast cells lining the stomach. The histamine then triggers a large acid outpouring, which can result in ulcer formation.

Small Intestine and Colon

Allergy to milk is a frequent cause of chronic duodenal ulcers and colitis. Whenever these conditions exist dairy products should be suspected. Allergy to grain, especially wheat, is another common precipitator of intestinal distress.

The Gall Bladder

Eating foods to which one is allergic can create gall bladder distress. The allergic reaction here causes swelling of the bile duct, which impairs emptying of the bile from the gall bladder into the small intestine. The accumulating fluid attracts infection and precipitates cholesterol, forming stones. Eggs have been shown to be the most common allergen affecting the gall bladder. Pork is also frequently involved, precipitating such severe symptoms that surgical removal of the gall bladder may result. In one study involving sixty-nine patients with gallstones, 92% reacted to egg, 63% reacted to pork, 52% reacted to onion, 34% reacted to fowl and 21% reacted to coffee.

The Pancreas

When food is eaten, one of the first organs to be affected is the pancreas. The pancreas reacts first with over-stimulation. When over-stimulation is sustained long enough, inhibition or decreased function results. Production of bicarbonate, the alkaline fluid that neutralizes the stomach acid in the small intestine, is the first function to suffer. When the stomach acid is not neutralized, acid can be absorbed through the intestine and create an over-acid condition in the body. A common symptom of acidity is headache.

The next function of the pancreas to be inhibited is the digestive enzyme production. These are the enzymes necessary to break down foods into absorbable products. A little-known function of proteolytic enzymes is that they also act as regulators of inflammatory reactions in the body. In other words, they can be used by the body to reduce or prevent inflammation. When proteolytic enzyme production is decreased, inflammatory kinins and prostaglandins can accumulate in ever-increasing quantity in the tissues, thus evoking inflammatory reactions throughout the body.

When not enough digestive enzymes are produced by the Pancreas, two major things happen. First, undigested fragments of food can be absorbed through the intestinal lining and into the blood stream. Antibodies recognize these particles as foreign invaders and attack them, creating allergic reactions within the body. The fewer enzymes, the more undigested food particles there are in the intestine. The higher the concentration of these particles in the intestine, the more particles can be absorbed into the blood.

Secondly, diminished enzyme output causes a lack of protein digestion; amino acids are the end products of protein digestion and when there are not enough proteolytic enzymes, the amino acid production suffers. Antibodies, hormones and enzymes are all built from amino acids. Insulin, needed for glucose metabolism, is made entirely from amino acids. The immune system is adversely affected due to lowered antibody production. Without sufficient amino acids, more digestive enzymes cannot be made, and a self-perpetuating, vicious cycle begins.

The last function of the pancreas to be affected by allergic reaction is insulin production. A lack of insulin is associated with diabetes.

The Blood Vessels

Food reactions often create vast changes in arteries. These changes include spasms, swelling and dilation. In the temporal arteries, food reactions often cause constriction and edema, resulting in migraine. Vascular spasms have been implicated in some cases of epilepsy. If the coronary arteries are involved allergically, damage to the lining may occur, leading to cholesterol accumulation and myocardial infarction (heart attack).

The Heart

The following symptoms have been seen in allergy affecting the heart: extra heartbeats, tachycardia (fast heartbeat), flutters, fibrillation, angina (pain), inflammation of the pericardium (sac surrounding the heart) and murmurs. These symptoms may result from allergic reactions to foods, tobacco, antibiotics or other drugs. 25% of arrhythmia is triggered by food allergies.

Hypoglycemia (low blood sugar)

Unstable blood sugar, or hypoglycemia, can cause a wide range of symptoms similar to allergy such as fatigue, overweight, light headedness, confusion, frequent hunger pains, anxiety, nervousness, weakness, panic attacks and depression. In his book *Victory Over Diabetes*, Dr. William H. Philpott states that both high and low blood sugar can be seen in a person who has eaten any food or come in contact with any chemical to which he reacts allergically. In other words, any substance that can elicit an allergic reaction in an individual will raise or lower blood sugar levels, evoking symptoms of hypoglycemia.

The problem is not the type of food, such as sugar, that has traditionally been restricted in the diet of the hypoglycemic, but with the allergic reaction to a specific chemical or food. Dr. Philpott cites the case of a man with diabetes. This example demonstrates that blood sugar levels can change dramatically due to contact with substances other than food!

I have observed for quite some time many diabetics who reacted very seriously to petrochemical hydrocarbons, such as found in exhaust fumes from cars, in perfumes or in fumes from natural gas. In Carl's case, a 30-minute test exposure to auto exhaust, as is usually experienced in city traffic, produced a shift in blood sugar from 40 milligrams % before exposure to well over a 180 milligrams % after exposure.

Obesity

Obesity usually involves addiction to several foods. Along with addictions come cravings and accompanying withdrawal effects. The foods you crave and eat the most often, or more than three times a week, are very likely to be your specific allergic foods. It is not a coincidence that the most frequently eaten foods are the most common allergens. Craving and insatiable hunger are characteristic symptoms of withdrawal. When the food is subsequently eaten, the person feels better – another tip-off of an addiction.

Addiction is also indicated by the fact that when foods are spaced out or rotated on the basis of once every four to five days, there is a startling reduction in the hunger urge. If you have a craving for something sweet, especially following a meal, your blood sugar has probably dropped due to an allergic reaction to something you just ate. The mere elimination of foods to which a person reacts allergically results in about ten pounds of weight loss with no other dietary change.

Another interesting fact concerns lipase, the enzyme that digests fat. The lipase levels of fat cells in an obese person are much lower than the lipase levels of fat cells of a normal-weight individual. Lipase is necessary in the cell for the cell's fat to be mobilized and subsequently burned for energy. This indicates that an obese person may have a lipase deficiency, or exhausted lipase production.

Musculoskeletal System

One of the more poorly recognized areas of allergy is its relation to the muscles and joints. Of all the muscle aches and pains, those in the muscles of the lower and upper back, neck and shoulders are especially linked to diet and maladaptive or allergic reactions. Dr. Rowe observed muscle aches and pains to be part of a syndrome that he called "allergic toxemia." The main symptoms he observed were fatigue and headaches, drowsiness, mental confusion, slowness of thought, irritability, depression and body aching.

Rowe was able to correlate specific foods to these symptoms. The patient may describe these symptoms as pulling and drawing sensations and stiffness or aching at the base of the neck. In the lower half of the body, the muscles most commonly affected are the hamstrings in the legs as well as the lower back muscles. Experiments have shown that these symptoms can all be reproduced by challenges with test foods or chemicals in susceptible persons. Instances of acute low back pain, acute bursitis and acute torticollis (stiff neck) are not uncommon. These aches, pains and stiffness are most common when a person first arises in the morning. If a person has recurring episodes, and is otherwise chronically ill, allergies should be investigated.

Arthritis (joints)

It is well established that joint symptoms do occur in people who have allergic symptoms. Dr. James C. Breneman found relief of arthritic symptoms in at least half of arthritic patients when their food allergens were identified and eliminated. Milk, wheat, egg, corn and pork were the most common food allergens. Doctors have long been aware of a relationship between gastrointestinal disease and arthritis. For example, a frequent side effect of intestinal bypass surgery is the development of a rheumatoid-type arthritis. Many gastrointestinal infections result in arthritis. Numerous studies show that arthritis can be produced at will in humans by feeding them foods to which they are allergic, and that the symptoms respond favorably when these foods are eliminated from the diet. It has been discovered that diet can precipitate arthritis in two ways: by either being deficient in nutrients, or by containing nutrients the body is not able to absorb and use. This paves the way for the second stage, allergic reactions.

The status of food allergy as a precipitative agent in rheumatoid arthritis has been demonstrated on numerous occasions since 1949. More recently, arthritis and environmental chemical pollutants have been investigated and have been found to have a high correlation. Theron G. Randolph, MD found that "with but rare exceptions, cases of rheumatoid arthritis now respond favorably to the avoidance of incriminated foods and chemical exposures including air pollutants, food and water additives and contaminants and synthetically derived or chemically contaminated drugs." He reports that when patients fasted and then were challenged with specific foods that symptoms developed.

A typical case from his report is given below, in which the patient fasted and then challenged with the following foods:

Apple	30 minutes	abdominal distress and arthritis
Cane sugar	15 minutes	Pains in knees and hands and abdominal cramps
Corn	10 minutes	severe arthritic pain
Lamb	35 minutes	severe arthritis
Orange	40 minutes	Intermittent waves of apprehension and depression followed by progressively severe arthritis

The January 1980 issue of *Annals of Allergy* reported a study involving subjects with both osteoarthritis and rheumatoid arthritis, the two main types of arthritic disease. 87% of the test subjects were found to have allergies that could cause such common symptoms as swelling and pain. Dr. James C. Breneman considers joint pain to be a very late manifestation of a food allergy reaction. He further states that, "The immunological etiology of arthritis seems well established." Part of the problem, he reports, is that often the joint pains may not appear for 42 to 72 hours after exposure to the allergic food. In the case of reaction to pork, symptoms may not appear for five days.

Upper Respiratory Infections

The nasal and sinus membranes are very sensitive to allergic irritants. These irritants do not have to be inhaled. They can also be foods to which a person is allergic. Once the membranes are irritated and swollen they are easily infected by bacteria or viruses, or they can become reactive to pollens and dust. These edematous tissues become chronically infected by repeated exposure to foods or inhalants that trigger allergic reactions.

Asthma (lungs)

Mast cells line the bronchi (the tubes leading from the trachea to the lungs). When the cells encounter an allergen, they release inflammatory products, which cause inflammation in the tissues. This irritation produces muscular contractions, which restrict airflow through the bronchial passage. Common irritants include tobacco smoke, chemical fumes, very cold air, bacterial infections, aspirin, sulfites and MSG (monosodium glutamate), but any food or air pollutant can be involved. The most common foods involved in asthma are milk, egg, wheat, seafood, peanuts and nuts.

Nephrosis (kidney disease)

Studies show that children with nephrosis are made significantly worse when fed their individual food allergens. Proteinuria (protein in the urine) improved when the allergens were eliminated from the diet.

Adrenal Glands

People exhibiting multiple allergies (30 or more), often have weakened adrenal glands. The adrenal glands are important because they produce hormones such as cortisone, which helps to prevent or decrease the intensity of allergic reactions. Excessive ingestion of white sugar and white flour products and other refined foods stress the adrenal glands. People with weakened adrenals tend to crave salt.

Headache

In cases where headaches are caused by allergenic foods, symptoms usually appear within an hour of consumption. Fatigue is considered the most frequent allergic symptom, however headache runs a close second. It makes more sense to investigate headache from the standpoint of its possible environmental cause than to treat it with painkillers. The most common foods reported to be involved in headache are milk, chocolate, peanuts, pork, egg and coffee. According to many researchers, food allergy is the number one cause of migraine headache. Leon Unger, MD and Joel Cristol, MD reported in their article *Allergic Migraines* which appeared in the *Annals of Allergy* that migraine headache is an allergic disease caused by one or more foods. Many prominent researchers have since supported this view.

Fatigue

Fatigue is the number one allergic sign. It tends to be worse in the morning and again in late afternoon. No amount of rest relieves the tiredness.

Diagnosing Allergy

Because of the widely varying manifestations of allergy in the many tissues of the body, developing valid tests for allergy, especially food allergy, has been a challenge. Zoltan P. Rona MD points out, "Since over 90% of all food allergies are of the delayed-onset type, skin tests and the IgE RAST will not detect the vast majority of food allergies. Nevertheless, conventional doctors continue to use them for that purpose and often conclude that the patient does not have any food allergies, even though no tests were ever done for delayed-hypersensitivity food reactions."

Many different diagnostic tests have been devised; all of which have their own strengths and weaknesses. Some of the more common tests used to detect allergy are described below.

Skin Testing

The basic method is pricking the skin to deliver a solution of allergen under the skin. The skin is then observed for various degrees of swelling and redness. While this is one of the most widely used tests to identify allergy, it works best for only certain types of allergy, especially inhalant allergy. Where food allergy is concerned, it may not produce a positive result simply because the required IgE antibody is not found in the skin. In this case, the IgE may be localized to some other tissue such as the intestine or nose, and it has not entered the general circulation (blood stream), which is the reason it is not present in the skin. It is known that the skin-scratch tests fail to detect 50% of food allergies.

RAST (Radioallergosorbent Test)

The RAST is a blood test which measures the number of IgE antibodies contained in it. It requires the presence of an IgE antibody to detect allergy. This test is more expensive to administer than skin testing. It is considered to be a good test for airborne allergens.

ELISA/ACT Test

The ELISA/ACT is a blood test that measures the presence of antibodies and abnormal white blood cell reactions to food. This test is capable of detecting delayed food allergies. IgG and IgG complex mediators are involved in 80% of all food allergy reactions. The ELISA test can detect both IgE and IgG mediated allergies.

Cytotoxic Test

This test observes the reactions of living white blood cells, red blood cells, and platelets when exposed to various foods and chemicals. When subsequent changes to the blood cells are observed, the test is considered positive for that food or chemical.

Elimination-Provocation

This test is the most widely accepted by the medical community. The patient either fasts on water only or is given a hypoallergenic diet for five days to one week. Then foods are reintroduced one at a time and the patient is observed for reactions (symptoms). The main disadvantage of this test is, of course, the time involved. It can take days or weeks. In addition, the symptoms produced do not necessarily distinguish between an actual allergic reaction and intolerance.

Sublingual Provocation

This test is performed by placing a test substance under the tongue. Then a major muscle is tested for a change in muscle strength. Weakening of the muscle when challenged with the test substance is an indication of sensitivity to that substance.

Dr. George Goodheart, the developer of applied kinesiology, pioneered the study of the connection between a substance placed under the patient's tongue and alterations in muscle strength. When an allergen or substance that an individual is sensitive to is placed in the mouth, there is an immediate and measurable weakening of that individual's muscle strength.

Dr. Hugh Cox, a founder of the British Society of Clinical Ecology, extended this work by taking a dilution of a food concentrate rather than the actual food, placing it under the patient's tongue and observing changes in muscle strength. In subsequent tests, he injected the dilution of the food concentrate under the skin to produce a skin reaction, such as a welt or flare on the skin surface. This is similar to the familiar skin prick test for allergy. Dr. Cox noticed that when the same dilution that caused a skin reaction was placed under the patient's tongue, it would produce dramatically weakened muscle responses. This is an objective and precise correlation between the two methods of testing. Dr. Cox further experimented by placing the drops on the skin itself. He got an identical weak muscle response. These weakened responses were later confirmed in double blind studies. Dr. Cox believes that when the body comes in contact with an allergen, the electrical potential of the allergen interferes with the electrical firing of the motor endplate of the muscle, thereby producing the muscle changes.

7

The Secret of Food Allergy

Do you crave a certain food frequently? Do you eat it even though you don't feel good the next day? Do you feel immediately better upon eating a certain food? If the answer is yes, you may be addicted. We tend to think of addiction in terms of substances such as drugs, caffeine, tobacco and alcohol. But is it possible to be addicted to foods such as wheat, cheese or pickles? What are the signs? Addiction goes hand in hand with allergy. With foods, addictions can be either conscious or subconscious. Your favorite foods are usually the ones to which you are allergic and also addicted.

Addiction causes chronic symptoms often hours or days after the food is eaten. Some of these symptoms include fatigue, weakness, headaches, irritability, and depression. When the addictive food is eaten again, the symptoms disappear temporarily. However, a person can often keep himself in a symptom-free state by eating the addictive food frequently, thereby postponing symptoms of withdrawal. The result is chronic stress to the body, eventually leading to chronic and degenerative disease.

The book *Clinical Ecology* reports that, "Food addiction has the same characteristics of relief on exposure and emergence of delayed reactions as has addiction to tobacco, narcotics or alcohol." It is possible to be addicted to anything, including common foods and chemicals such as in perfume and hair spray.

Foods are the primary potential addictant for three reasons:
1. The sheer bulk of food – large amounts are eaten; two to five pounds per day.
2. Frequency – food is eaten daily, several times a day.

3. Intimacy or duration of exposure - food stays in contact with the digestive tract for a long time.

Withdrawal reactions last four to five days when an addictive food is removed from the diet. Eating the food after withholding it from the diet for four to five days will cause an increased allergic reaction. This is the basis for using the elimination diet as a diagnostic test.

Four Cardinal Signs of Addiction:

1. Obsession: The person often cannot stop thinking about food. He or she plans the next time he will eat it. When he is close to getting the food, he may feel an anxiety or excitement that does not let up until actually eating the food. He or she arranges their life in ways that will facilitate obtaining the food.

2. Negative consequences: The person will eat the food, in spite of the fact that it may have negative consequences. For instance, a person eats six candy bars even though he knows he will feel bloated, tired and unable to do more than watch television that evening. Addictive behaviors produce pleasure, relief and other payoffs that ignore harmful consequences.

3. Lack of control: Do you know anyone who, once he eats the first doughnut, cannot stop until the whole box is gone? Or eats one potato chip and cannot stop until the whole bag is empty? Inability to control or stop the behavior is a mark of addiction. When the person tries to bring the behavior under control, willpower alone is not enough. The food is controlling the person, rather than the other way around.

4. Denial: Denying that a food can be the cause of your burning stomach, aching shoulders or swollen joints is characteristic of addiction. You dismiss obvious symptoms by saying, "I didn't eat very much of it," or, "My doctor says it can't possibly be the cause of my colitis," or by avoiding the subject altogether.

Why, you might wonder, are the most commonly eaten foods such as milk, wheat, egg and corn also the foods most frequently found to be allergenic? The answer lies in understanding enzyme deficiency. When you eat a food frequently, such as milk on your breakfast cereal, a glass of milk for lunch, an ice cream cone in the afternoon and milk in the form of cheese on your pizza for dinner, you are calling on specific enzymes to digest that milk. When this eating pattern continues over days, weeks and years, you may create an enzyme deficiency for that food. The same is true for wheat. When you eat wheat in the form of toast or pancakes or doughnuts for breakfast, wheat in the bread of your sandwich for lunch and wheat in dinner rolls or in breaded entrees in the evening, specific enzymes are called on over and over until they are eventually depleted. Milk and wheat are the two most common allergenic foods and they are often eaten together; cereal and milk, cheese sandwich, cheeseburger with a glass of milk and pizza with a wheat crust and cheese, are common examples. This stresses the enzyme systems even more.

Anything consumed on a daily basis is a potential allergen. Corn is another good example. A person may not eat corn itself, but may still be consuming great quantities of corn daily in the form of corn oil, cornstarch, corn syrup, cereal, dextrin, corn meal or alcohol made from corn. By 1967, 130 supermarket products contained some form of corn.

All chemical and ingested food allergies and addictions eventually lead to pancreatic injury. With a compromised pancreas, production of bicarbonate needed to neutralize stomach acid and for the production of enzymes, are the most affected. Through allergy and addiction, foods can harm your health over a period of time.

The Difference between Allergy and Addiction

Clinical Ecology states, Allergic and allergic-like maladaptive reactions have been so characterized by the fact that immediate and/or relatively immediate reactions occur on exposure. Addiction has been characterized by an initial relief, or partial relief, on exposure and the emergence of delayed reactions which can again be relieved by exposure.

Common Withdrawal Symptoms from Food

1. Influenza-like feelings
2. Aching of all parts of the body
3. High temperature or fever
4. Severe headaches
5. Palpitations
6. Pains in parts of the body that have not been affected before

Withdrawal effects have been known to persist as long as 20 hours when an allergic food is eaten only once in 24 hours. When the allergic food is eaten three times a day, symptoms are most likely to be noticed first thing upon arising in the morning.

It is easier to become addicted to a refined, processed food than to a whole food in its natural state. A refined food has lost its normal protective ratios of synergistic vitamins, minerals and enzymes either by removal or destruction. This alters the way the refined food is metabolized in the body. For example, sugar acts more like a drug in the body than like a food because it has been refined to a pure form, devoid of its complementary nutrients. In its natural state, as sugar cane, it supplies B vitamins and many trace minerals including chromium.

When refined sugar is eaten, these nutrients must be supplied from body stores in order for the sugar to be metabolized. If these nutrient stores are depleted, alternate metabolic pathways of the body must be used, which can create an imbalance in the body's biochemistry. This imbalance results in altered signals to the brain, leading to craving and addiction. Eating whole foods in a natural state has been shown clinically to be the quickest way to eliminate cravings.

Understanding Food Allergy

Food allergy is far more common than generally accepted. For doctors who do not work in the allergy field, it is popular to sit back and dismiss this idea. However, those health care professionals who have had first-hand experience with patients are beginning to relate a different story, especially when their patients respond dramatically well to an allergy protocol. These doctors are finding that the effects of food allergy are not limited to just the air passages, the skin, and the digestive tract. Although these are frequent sites, it has been shown that allergens can enter the bloodstream, travel throughout the body show up anywhere the blood flows. It has further been shown that these effects produce a wide variety of physical and mental symptoms.

Because most food allergens cause delayed reactions, which may occur anywhere from hours to five days after ingestion of the food, and account for about 95% of adverse food reactions, the connection of the food to the reaction is often overlooked by both the allergic person and the attending doctor. These delayed reactions are harder to detect and many of the usual tests to diagnose airborne allergens do not apply well to food allergens. According to James Braly, MD,

> Delayed food allergy appears to be simply the inability of your digestive tract to prevent large quantities of partially digested and undigested food from entering the bloodstream. Once in the bloodstream, allergens may be deposited in tissue, causing the symptoms and inflammatory diseases we call by other names.

Food Allergy and the Immune System

Because people with food allergies generally have incompetent digestive tracts, they are unable to absorb, transport, and utilize foods properly for nutrition. This causes varying degrees of malnutrition and affects the immune system in two different ways.

1. The immune system relies on nutrients for its protective activities. When it becomes nutrient depleted, it is unable to maintain a high degree of protection for the body. As a consequence, the functions of the immune system become slowly more and more impaired.
2. When incompletely digested food enters the bloodstream, the white blood cells of the immune system are called upon to finish the job of digestion. The white blood cells have not only the responsibility for destroying the products of poor digestion, but also T-cell defense against foreign invaders, clean-up of inflammatory debris and removal of damaged cells and immune complexes. The leukocytes (white blood cells) are normally rich in enzymes and it is by enzymatic activity that the leukocytes are able to finish digestion not completed inside the intestine.

The combination of fewer nutrients available for the immune system, and the consequent increased workload of the influx of allergic substances, affects the functions of the immune system, which begins to wear down. Over time, these functions become more and more impaired and the allergic person can become significantly more prone to other diseases.

The Difference between Airborne Allergy and Food Allergy

Airborne allergy is the allergy that we are all most familiar with and the easiest to diagnose. When an unfamiliar substance (such as pollens, dust, molds), enters the body for the first time, the body begins the process of manufacturing antibodies specific to that substance. These IgE antibodies will be ready to act the next time the substance is encountered. Meanwhile they attach themselves to mast cells of the immune system. Tens of millions of these mast cells line the air passages, skin, digestive tract and small blood vessels throughout the body. Each mast cell is coated with hundreds of thousands of IgE antibodies. When the allergen again enters the body and is exposed to these IgE coated mast cells, an allergic reaction occurs releasing inflammatory substances and triggering a cascade of allergic symptoms such as watering eyes, runny nose, sinus congestion and pain, itching, rash, wheezing.

Recently, another type of mast cell has been recognized. This type of mast cell resides in the connective tissue lining of the intestinal tract. Instead of IgE antibody being produced when a food allergen is ingested, a free-floating antibody called secretory IgA is released into the digestive tract. Secretory IgA coats the particles of the offending food entering the small intestine from the stomach. When a food allergen and the secretory IgA antibody combine, it stimulates the secretion of a thick, protective mucus coating along the mucosal lining of the intestine. Then, as the allergic food chemically bonds with the mast-cell antibodies specific to it, powerful chemicals are suddenly released. These chemicals may include histamine, bradykinin, inflammatory prostaglandins, leukotrienes, heparin, serotonin, and others. Although an allergic reaction has just occurred, it has followed a different pathway in the body and used different chemicals than the airborne reaction.

However, the food allergen reaction is more insidious than the airborne reaction. Whereas the airborne reaction is fairly local (eyes, nose, sinuses, air passages), the food allergen reaction has far-reaching consequences. For example, the released inflammatory prostaglandins cause the stomach to secrete less hydrochloric acid. Hydrochloric acid is necessary to stimulate the production of pepsinogen, a protein-digesting enzyme. Without sufficient pepsinogen, protein cannot be properly digested. This lessened production of hydrochloric acid also causes the food to enter the small intestine in an under acid state. Without sufficient acid, the pancreas under produces the bicarbonate necessary to alkalinize the food since it depends on the acid to stimulate this production. With less bicarbonate, the pancreas is also not stimulated to produce and release the necessary digestive enzymes to complete digestion. Paradoxically, because the food is not alkalinized, the original underacidic food now remains in a relative overacidic state in the small intestine.

The powerful chemicals released during the allergic reaction cause other serious problems. They are capable of causing inflammation of the intestine, which in turn will cause the intestine to become more permeable to the food particles, allowing more incompletely digested particles to gain entrance to the bloodstream. The healthy intestinal wall is a 1/8-inch thick mucosal membrane, which normally allows only fully digested food to proceed through to the bloodstream. When this lining becomes inflamed, its normal function is compromised and allergens can enter the blood and be carried to other parts of the body, creating further reactions in tissues throughout the body.

The Secret

Herein lies the secret of food allergy: When food is completely digested, that is, broken down to the smallest particle that it was designed to break down to, it is basically rendered non-allergic. This is because when food is fully digested and enters the bloodstream in that state, the immune system recognizes it as a familiar particle – food. When incompletely digested particles enter the bloodstream, the immune system recognizes them not as food, but as foreign invaders which provoke an attack (reaction). The secret to stopping food allergy then is to make sure that food is fully digested in order for the adverse reactions to stop.

Hugh A Sampson, MD, in the *Journal of the American College of Nutrition* (Volume 9, #4, 1990), states that, "The development of food allergy is the result of an interaction between food allergens, the gastrointestinal tract and the immune system."

Further proof that faulty digestion and allergic reactions are inter-twined is found in the textbook *Human Nutrition* which states: "Any major alteration of the molecular structure usually results in loss of allergic potential, thus digestion with the attendant splitting of the molecules into peptides and amino acids renders the protein non-al-lergic, depending on the extent of the hydrolytic degradation."

Intestinal Permeability, Acquired CHO Intolerance, published by John Hopkins University Press in 1981, states that, "Increased macromolecular absorption may lead to the development of hyper-sensitivity and allergy to foodstuffs in the susceptible host."

Why Avoidance is Not the Answer

The usual advice given to a person with allergies is to avoid the al-lergic substance. This does tend to bring some amount of relief to the allergy sufferer, but it can also seriously limit one's lifestyle. While you are staying indoor to avoid pollen and dust, and keeping your humid-ifier clean; scouring the bedroom for dust mites; laundering daily with hot water; checking your potted plants for mold and mildew; decont-aminating your kitchen, and getting rid of your pets, other people are going about their business, leading full lives. All of these activities may make you feel better, but they will not get you well. In most cases it is just not possible to avoid all the possible allergic triggers.

If you have had allergy skin testing performed, you probably test-ed positive for yeast and mold. Avoiding yeast, fungus and mold is nearly impossible because fungal spores are everywhere. They are in every breath you take. Fungus has been found 11,000 feet in the air and 5,000 feet under the ground. Mold has been found growing in-side the gasoline tank of the wings of jet aircraft. No matter how clean you keep your home, yeast and mold still thrive. If you put un-covered cultured Petri dishes in each room of your house, fungus will be growing in them within 24 hours.

All of the focus of avoidance advice has been on the external envi-ronment. It is time to turn our attention to the internal environ-ment. What is the difference between an allergy sufferer and a healthy individual? The difference is what is going on inside the body. Both people are exposed to the external environment, but only one of them is reacting adversely to it. Therefore it is not the external environment that is the cause, but rather something that is going on inside the body of the allergy sufferer.

Rotation of foods is another form of avoidance. By eating each food only once every 4 to 5 days, many adverse reactions can be avoided. This may make you feel better, but it again does make you well. We know this from the fact that when you stop rotating the foods, many of the symptoms begin to return. Rotating foods month after month can become a cumbersome lifestyle. Rotating foods is a control mechanism because all foods cannot be eliminated for long periods of time and rotation of foods helps control symptoms by controlling exposure.

Elimination is also a form of avoidance. Most people think that if they are allergic to something, they are allergic to it for life and the substance must be eradicated from their lives for good. This is simply not true. When conditions inside the body (which produced the allergy) change, the allergic symptoms will change.

Desensitization can also help allergy symptoms. Starting with tiny amounts of substance and gradually increasing those amounts can help train the body not to react to the substance. However, this also does not take into account conditions inside the body that may be producing the allergy in the first place. While the person may stop reacting to the substance that was desensitized, he or she often starts reacting to new substances. Food allergy especially tends to rotate into new foods. This is because desensitization does nothing to help heal the digestive tract.

Intestinal Permeability

The gastrointestinal lining is supposed to absorb nutrients and at the same time act as a barrier to toxins. Intestinal permeability is a clinical disorder in which the basic defect is an intestinal lining that is more permeable than normal. This allows food particles, bacteria and other organisms and/or their toxins access to the bloodstream and other parts of the body. After lying dormant for a number of years, it is refreshing to see new laboratory studies being conducted on this extremely important and key element to healing allergies and many other chronic disorders.

65

The phrase, *leaky gut syndrome* is often used instead of the more correct term increased intestinal permeability. It is a condition, rather than a disease or illness but, once developed, it can lead to many other disorders. In fact, people with leaky gut syndrome often display a wide variety of symptoms ranging from arthritis, chronic fatigue, irritable bowel syndrome, and all sorts of allergies including food allergies.

Why Is The Intestinal Barrier So Important?

A healthy intestine does more than just digest food. It is an immune barrier that protects the body from foreign invaders. A healthy intestinal lining allows only properly digested fats, proteins and starches to pass through so that they can be assimilated. At the same time it also provides a barrier to keep out unwanted, undigested molecules, bacterial products, and other foreign substances. In between the cells of the intestine are normally tight fitting junctions which do not allow large molecules to pass through. However, when this area becomes irritated or inflamed, these junctions between the cells loosen up and permit larger molecules to pass through. The immune system interprets these large molecules as foreign invaders and this stimulates an antibody reaction. Some of the substances that may pass through a damaged intestinal lining are bacteria and fungus, toxic molecules including those produced by the process of digestion, and undigested food particles. These may pass directly through the weakened junctions and into the bloodstream.

Protection by this immune barrier is supplied by a number of mechanisms including:

1. The intestinal mucosa (physical barrier)
2. Intestinal secretions (an example is secretory IgA antibodies)
3. Lymphocytes (white blood cells)

The intestine can be considered an immune barrier with some doctors considering it the body's first line of defense. When the intestine fails to do its job, adverse immune reactions can develop.

According to Sherry Rogers MD, in *Townsend Letter for Doctors*, 1995,

> The Leaky Gut Syndrome or LGS is a poorly recognized, but extremely common problem. It is rarely tested for. Basically, it repre-

sents a hyper-permeable intestinal lining. In other words, large spaces develop between the cells of the gut wall, and bacteria, toxins, and foods leak in.

Zoltan P. Rona MD states in Childhood Illness and the Allergy Connection, 1997:

The Leaky Gut Syndrome is a very common problem and rapidly increasing, especially in children suffering from recurrent infections of any kind who are constantly on antibiotics. Leaky gut syndrome is at least as common as all the immune system diseases put together.

Conditions Produced by Leaky Gut (Increased Intestinal Permeability)

1 Fatigue
2 Allergies and food intolerance
3 Joint Pains (arthritis)
4 Muscle pains
5 Abdominal pain
6 Diarrhea
7 Rashes
8 Abdominal distension
9 Poor memory
10 Shortness of breath
11 Chemical intolerance
12 Fevers of unknown origin
13 Environmental illness
14 Intestinal infections
15 Pancreatic insufficiency
16 Eczema
17 Childhood hyperactivity

Diseases Associated with Leaky Gut (Increased Intestinal Permeability)

Acne
Alcoholism
Ankylosing spondylitis
Arthritis (some types of chronic)
Autoimmune disease
Celiac disease
Childhood hyperactivity
Colitis
Crohn's disease
Cystic fibrosis
Eczema
Environmental illness
Fibromyalgia (contributes to)
Inflammatory bowel disease
Irritable bowel syndrome
Liver dysfunction
Multiple food and chemical
  sensitivities
Pancreatic insufficiency
Psoriasis
Urticaria

Wanda's Success Story; Revived Back to Life

Modern medicine is where we have been trained to look for help, but hopefully, after I share my story, you will see there are other alternatives, healthier alternatives out there.

I was never a healthy child. I had severe allergies and no matter what I did, I just kept deteriorating. By the time I was 16, I went to a medical allergist who told me that by the time I was 30, I would be dead for I would be allergic to myself. Year after year, specialist after specialist, I kept deteriorating. I was diagnosed with the beginning of multiple sclerosis, Lupus, chronic fatigue syndrome and fibromyalgia. By age 25, my outlook on life was bleak. I had no energy. I was physically disabled. I had lost feeling on my left side. I had seen a chronic fatigue specialist, a rheumatologist, a neurologist, an allergist, and a lung specialist. Here was their advice. "Wanda, you are young. Go home and learn to live with it; we can't help you." The day I heard these words was the day I lost hope. Anyone knows that the worst thing that can happen to a person is to lose hope, for once hope is gone, your will to survive leaves too.

If there is one message I would like to impart, it is this – THERE IS ALWAYS HOPE. From a friend, I was told of Dr. Carolee Bateson-Koch. I attended her lecture and thought, "Wanda, what do you have to lose?" Nothing - that was the answer, so in April of 1995, I made an appointment with Dr. Bateson-Koch. This appointment not only gave me hope, but a new life.

Boy, was I sick, but here is the best part – I was curable. Yes, the multiple sclerosis symptoms showed up as did the chronic fatigue, systemic candidiasis, weakened organs, indications of worms, parasites and about twenty allergies. I was so desperate for help I never once complained about what I had to take, or the diet I needed to be on to become healthy. Hey, after all, what is six weeks of your life on a natural plan, compared to a lifetime of being ill?

I am happy to report that one year after beginning Dr. Carolee's program, I am still free of symptoms. This certainly is a far cry from the "learn how to live with it" advice. I didn't have to learn to live with it, I had to learn to try something new. I had to learn about natural medicine.

I now work full-time and still have extra energy to do the things I enjoy. I am now 30, alive, and feel like I have been given the kiss of life to replace the kiss of death that I had previously received. I certainly can never thank Dr. Bateson-Koch enough for her knowledge, expertise and care. Without these things, I would be buried today (at least that's what the doctors told me).

How Does the Gut Become Leaky?

The intestinal lining becomes leaky by inflammation. Once the gut lining becomes inflamed or damaged, the function is disrupted. The spaces between the cells of the lining enlarge, allowing large protein molecules and other substances to be absorbed through the normally small spaces between the gut lining cells.

Intestinal inflammation can be caused by any of the following or their combinations:

1. Infections such as bacteria, fungal, viral, or parasitic. These organisms create tissue damage directly or by the toxins that they excrete.
2. Drugs, particularly antibiotics, birth-control pills, NSAIDS (non-steroidal anti-inflammatory drugs such as aspirin and ibuprofen), cytotoxic drugs, corticosteroids, alcohol and caffeine.
3. Allergic reactions along the intestinal lining created by foods and beverages and/or various chemicals added to foods and beverages.
4. Nutritional deficiencies created by diets high in sugar and refined foods.
5. Incomplete digestion
6. Heightened exposure to environmental toxins
7. Stress

How is Intestinal Permeability Corrected?

The key to healing the intestinal lining lies in following three steps.

1. Rid the digestive system of all known stresses such as unfavorable bacteria, fungus, food allergens, chemicals and other irritants.
2. Repair the intestinal lining using proper diet, herbs and supplements.
3. Replace (reculture) the beneficial colon bacteria using probiotic supplements and diet.

The Three Most Commonly Overlooked Conditions Leading to Allergy

1. Yeasts and Molds
2. Parasites
3. Digestive Difficulties

Although each person is unique in their individual symptoms, there are nevertheless common similarities, which emerge and become evident over the course of many years when thousands of people have been treated. These similarities become an observable basic underlying pattern that characterizes most of allergy. In other words, a very high percentage of people with allergies tend to have these three common and usually overlooked conditions which lead to their present state. Conversely, when these three conditions are removed, or improved, much of their allergic symptoms disappear.

8

The First Common Condition Leading to Allergy: Yeasts and Molds

In addition to understanding of how allergy arises, affects tissues, is recognized and what symptoms it can produce, there are other factors that dramatically affect allergy. Although breathing in yeast and mold spores can trigger symptoms, yeast and mold actually exert their worst effects by producing infection within the body. Infections by yeast and mold have an important connection to allergy and are frequently found in individuals suffering from allergy.

Candida albicans is by far the most common opportunistic yeast involved in allergic symptoms. In fact, when Candida is present as a systemic infection, it is virtually impossible for a person to recover from allergy until the Candida infection is brought under control.

Candida albicans, a yeast-like fungus, normally exists in small colonies in the intestinal tract of healthy individuals along with beneficial bacteria and other microbes. In this balanced state, it does not cause illness. However, if this balance is disrupted, Candida may multiply rapidly, invade other tissues and become an overgrowth that is capable of causing, contributing, or exacerbating chronic conditions, as well as serious disease. Candidiasis is also known as a polysymptomatic disease, which means that a person will exhibit a whole list of symptoms, many of which may seem bizarre. The afflicted person may be labeled as neurotic or a hypochondriac. In the last ten years, a great deal of research has emerged and helped to create a better understanding of Candida and its relationship to allergic disease.

Candidiasis Symptoms

The symptoms of candidiasis vary widely and are manifested throughout the body.

Digestive system - may exhibit bloating, gas, cramps, or irritable bowel syndrome

Nervous system - fatigue, anxiety, mood swings, "brain fog", depression, poor memory, and headaches. Candidiasis is strongly associated with learning disabilities and hyperactivity in children.

Skin - eczema, rash, acne and nail infections

Genitourinary - recurrent bladder and vaginal infections, genital rashes, prostatitis, rectal itching

Hormonal system - produces hormone-like substances that disrupt estrogen and interfere with hormonal communication.

Musculoskeletal - pain and swelling in the joints, vague aches and pains throughout the body.

Other symptoms commonly produced in conjunction with chronic candidiasis include the following: allergies, sinusitis, recurrent sore throat and ear infections, and sick all over feelings.

Symptoms tend to worsen on damp, rainy days and in places where molds can be inhaled. Symptoms may also intensify when candidiasis is combined with breathing in chemicals such as tobacco, smoke, perfumes, car exhaust and other pollutants.

When the normal ratio of yeast to friendly bacteria in the colon is disrupted, Candida albicans begins to grow and produce substances to enhance its environment. Candidiasis begins when the yeast gains access to the bloodstream and lymphatics. It has the ability to change from a single cell yeast into a pathological branching fungal form, which can multiply rapidly. It uses its root-like tentacles to perforate the intestinal wall, damaging cells. Eventually the organism may pass through the intestinal wall, gaining entrance to the bloodstream and lymphatics where either it or its toxins may travel to other parts of the body. Pathologists studying Candida albicans have discovered tiny abscesses throughout the body which consist of Candida albicans surrounded by a fibrin (a protein able to clot) and a connective tissue shell. This shell isolates Candida from being eliminated by the immune system. Symptoms created by this organism have been linked to all parts of the body.

Tony's Success Story

Tony, aged seven, weighed only 38 pounds and had not gained weight for several months. When I first saw him in my office, he displayed eczema, which had been on his arms and legs since birth. He had frequent nosebleeds, gas, and infections and was listless. He was also still wetting his bed at night.

Upon testing, Tony was found to be reactive to milk, sugar, yeast and grain dust. His pituitary, thymus and pancreas were stressed and underactive. His mother had taken him for numerous medical examinations with no results. The only medication he was receiving was a cortisone ointment that his mother said was not helping.

Findings from Tony's case history, examination and testing suggested this patient had been born with systemic Candida infection, which led to the multiplicity of his problems. He was put on a program to correct this condition and given Lactobacillus acidophilus to reculture his colon. He received chiropractic adjustments, nutritional plant enzymes and nutrient supplements to strengthen his immune system. The allergenic foods were eliminated from his diet.

Within two weeks, there was marked improvement in the eczema. Where the sores had been oozing red and raised above the skin level, they were now less red, flush with the skin, and did not itch. One month later, Tony was free of the eczema except for a small spot inside each elbow. The nosebleeds and bed-wetting had ceased.

However, at about this time, Tony developed a fever and swollen testicles. He was given antibiotics under medical therapy. The rash returned on his legs. When the course of antibiotics ran out, nutritional therapy was continued and the rash again disappeared. One year later, all symptoms were still gone and Tony had gained 15 pounds. He was now eating all foods except milk.

Established factors which lead to a pathological growth of Candida include the following:
- Drug therapy, particularly antibiotics, birth control pills, corticosteroids, and immunosuppressants
- Lowered immunity
- Mold in the environment
- High-sugar diets
- Candida may be acquired from birth from an infected mother

Of these factors, antibiotics has been the most implicated because of the ability of antibiotics to destroy up to 95% of the healthy colon microflora which keep yeast numbers in balance, thus allowing Candida to flourish. It is the intestinal flora that directly restricts the growth of Candida or its conversion to a pathological colony. These friendly bacteria keep Candida in balance by competing for food and by producing the B vitamin, biotin, which helps to block yeast overgrowth.

United States statistics show that in 1994, antibiotic prescriptions for humans numbered 281 million, or 15% of all prescriptions written. According to a US Food and Drug Administration Press Office publication, *Yeast Infection*, 1990, since 1950 "the increasing use of antibiotics, contraceptive hormones, corticosteroids and immunosuppressant drugs in medical practice has encouraged the growth of this yeast in many individuals." When corticosteroids are introduced, Candida may readily bind to the steroid molecule causing it to form budding hyphae (the branching tendrils and filaments). These filaments form an enzyme known as phospholipase at their tips which allows the filament to penetrate cellular walls. The action of this enzyme produces peroxide as a byproduct which can create localized inflammation along the gut wall and also, skin rashes.

Some people are sure that they have not taken antibiotics in any great amount. However, antibiotics are often present in today's meat supply. Almost all poultry, 70% of cattle and 90% of pigs raised commercially in the United States are ingesting antibiotics with their feed. There is evidence that some residues of these antibiotics remain in the meat and are transferable to humans when the meat is eaten.

How many individuals may be affected by abnormal Candida growth? No one knows for sure, but current estimates are that 35% of the general population may be affected by an overgrowth of Candida. However, the number escalates above 80% in individuals with allergies.

Just as Candida masquerades under a plethora of symptoms, it has also been given many names. Candida may be called candidiasis, systemic candidiasis, Candida related complex, chronic Candida syndrome, Candida albicans systemic overgrowth, candidiasis hypersensitivity, or mold, fungus, and intestinal yeast infection. The important distinction is that Candida may exist as a benign, universally present form of yeast in the normal gastrointestinal tract or, given the right conditions, it can exist as invasive intestinal candidiasis. It is in the latter form that it is capable of producing or contributing to the seemingly perplexing variety of symptoms.

Candida may spread throughout the body in a number of ways. For example, yeast organisms may spread out from the bowel to colonize the entire digestive tract, including the stomach, especially in individuals with low hydrochloric acid. Yeast may also colonize into the throat, mouth, and nasal passages, and down into the lungs. Candida may perforate the intestinal wall with its tiny, root-like structures called pseudomycelia. This perforation is a major mechanism seen in food allergy and food intolerance. It also allows intestinal toxins to leak into the bloodstream. In addition, by burrowing into the intestinal wall, this invasive form of yeast may trigger an inflammatory immune system condition in the intestinal wall itself. The perforation may ultimately lead to Candida passing through the intestinal wall and travelling in the bloodstream to other parts of the body. The fact that Candida can pass through the intestinal wall, accessing the bloodstream, was documented in a study in which a researcher ingested 80 grams. of Candida albicans. Fungus cells were later cultured from blood samples taken after three and six hours. Fungus cells were also cultured from urine samples taken after two and three hours.

Leo Galland, MD, collected data on 91 patients with candidiasis and compiled the following results:

91% reported fatigue
86% reported food intolerance
81% reported gastrointestinal disturbances
71% reported alcohol intolerance

61% reported chronic vaginitis
55% reported poor memory
54% reported depression
46% reported chemical hypersensitivity
44% reported PMS
39% reported anxiety
29% reported headaches
19% reported carbohydrate cravings

How is Candidiasis Diagnosed?

Virtually every healthy person carries the Candida organism in his or her intestinal tract. Because of this, many health care professionals feel that laboratory tests such as blood cultures and smears and stool analysis are not reliable ways to determine if there is an overgrowth of the fungus. Even if the stool culture is positive, there is not necessarily agreement among professionals as to the meaning of the results. Because laboratory tests are somewhat controversial, many experts in the field such as John Parks Trowbridge MD and William Crook MD, feel that Candida can be successfully diagnosed and treated without laboratory tests. A clinical diagnosis of candidiasis can be based on a self-administered questionnaire, personal history, physical examination, clinical tests of choice and the patient's response to a therapeutic Candida treatment program. To support this view, a study published in the summer, 1990, in *The Journal of Advancement of Medicine 3*, no. 2, was titled *An Evaluation of Self-Administered Questionnaires as an Aid in Diagnosis of Candida-Related-Complex.* The results of this study showed that three of the four different questionnaires tested proved to be equally as accurate in diagnosing Candida as laboratory blood tests, cultures, and antibody assays. In fact, some of the laboratory tests such as the *Candida Immuno Assay* and the *Albicans Antibody Titre Test* also require correlation to a questionnaire.

How is Candida Linked to Allergy?

The IgE antibody is considered a classic marker of allergy. It has been found that individuals with systemic candidiasis have an average of nearly a 2000% increase in IgE to Candida. Various studies have noted that many patients given antifungal drugs also have environmental allergies. Other studies demonstrate that patients with elevated IgE levels to Candida were also elevated to other antigens.

A minimum of 80 known toxins is secreted by pathogenic colonies of Candida and the body will respond by creating a specific antibody to each one. This stimulates non-specific symptoms that are often difficult to diagnose and easily misdiagnosed. For example, symptoms in the colon may be labeled with a general title like irritable bowel syndrome or regional enteritis when the symptoms may actually be inflammation caused by Candida. The patient may then be treated with a corticosteroid, which may decrease the inflammation but result in a dramatic increase in the Candida colonies.

According to recent research, Candida overgrowth manifests first in gastrointestinal and urinary tract disorders, then as allergic reactions. As the pathogenic organism continues to increase in the body, mental and emotional disturbances emerge followed by endocrine system compromise and eventual exhaustion.

Dr. William Crook remarks in his book, *Nature's Own Candida Cure* that, "Almost without exception, every person with a yeast-related problem is bothered by food sensitivities." Sensitivities, of course, can mean either food allergy or intolerance.

Andrew Wm. Sereda, MD echoes this view linking Candida with allergies in his book *The Many Faces of Yeast.* Dr. Sereda states," A common element of chronic candidiasis is the prominence of coexisting allergic symptoms. Hay fever, asthma, eczema, conjunctivitis and iritis, food allergies and at times very troublesome environmental allergic states may be present."

The Role of Candida in Food Allergy

Food allergy commonly occurs when incompletely digested food is able to enter the body through an inflamed intestinal barrier. These food molecules, unrecognized by the immune system as normal food because they are not in their fully digested state, trigger a variety of immune system reactions. Environmental chemicals and intestinal toxins may accompany the food through the malfunctioning intestinal barrier, increasing the complexity of possible interactions. When large Candida colonies are present along with inadequate beneficial flora in the intestines, alcohol and gas containing hydrocarbons may be produced. These substances may then accompany undigested food through the inflamed intestinal barrier and into the bloodstream, encouraging allergic reactions.

Lawrence A Plumlee, MD, has noted that when Candida toxins enter the bloodstream, the immune system overreacts to them, causing new food allergies to develop. The immune system changes, stimulated by the fungi, often result in problematic food and chemical sensitivities.

Laboratory studies done on rats indicate that Candida glycoproteins can stimulate histamine release from mast cells. Histamine is the main inflammatory product seen in allergies. Histamine creates membrane permeability and when histamine is released on a continual basis, it can be carried throughout the body, affecting distant tissues.

Joan's Success Story

Joan, age 25, was bothered by her hair falling out, creating a thin patch of on one side of her head. She also had pain in her right hip and lower abdomen. She was taking birth control pills, B vitamins and calcium.

Examination revealed that Joan had blood sugar instability and systemic Candida overgrowth. She was intolerant of wheat, milk, fish, shellfish, nuts and cheese. Although she was supplementing with calcium, she was deficient in both calcium and magnesium. She also had a copper toxicity.

Joan appeared to be experiencing an inflammatory kinin reaction in her right lower abdomen whenever she ate meat. This reaction was also causing pain in her right hip. Enzyme therapy resolved this situation within two weeks. She was put on a program to clear up the Candida overgrowth infection and reduce the copper toxicity. She was also given trace minerals and vitamins A, C and E. She received chiropractic adjustments to help strengthen and balance her structure and weak organs.

Most of Joan's symptoms cleared up within the first three weeks. However, her program was continued for three months to give all the tissues time to heal and strengthen, and to prevent recurrence. After that time, Joan did not require nutrient supplements. She also discontinued her birth control pills as she felt that they had contributed to her Candida infection.

Little-known Facts about Candida

- Researchers have discovered that Candida is not only able to change to a pathogenic form, it is capable of changing back again to its original shape. It has at least 17 variations, which allow it to elude the immune system and resist antifungal medications.
- Diets high in sugar and processed food favor Candida growth.
- Chlorine added to tap water can be toxic to friendly colon bacteria, thus indirectly favoring Candida growth.
- When Candida migrates to other tissues, it can grow unchecked and produce toxins that have systemic effects. These toxins are often capable of suppressing and inhibiting the immune system.
- Acetylaldehyde produced by Candida is able to suppress the T-cells (fighter cells) of the immune system, increase vascular permeability, enhance histamine release, and produce central nervous system symptoms through its interference with nerve transmissions. When acetylaldehyde is present, red blood flexibility is lost which decreases the rate at which red blood cells can carry oxygen to the tissues. Because the brain is very oxygen-dependent, central nervous system symptoms result. Mood swings, irritability, behavioral changes and headaches are common symptoms of central nervous system involvement.
- Candida has been shown to be able to convert the mercury vapor from mercury in silver amalgam dental fillings to methyl mercury. Studies indicate that mercury can be retained in brain tissue for 18 to 22 years.
- A common sign of Candida infection is intolerance to cheese, beer, wine and perfumes. Obvious reactions to these products are classical signs of Candida overgrowth.
- Babies can be born with Candida infection since the organism can cross the placental barrier in utero.
- Yeast cells produce hormone-like substances which stimulate

estrogen production in the body. In this way yeast cells can interfere with normal hormonal communication, causing inappropriate signals to be sent.

- Some reports indicate that Candida also produces alcohol in the system. People in whom this occurs may appear to be drunk or mentally confused without ever taking a drink.
- Candida is a polyantigenic organism. This means there have been 80 immunological allergic characteristics isolated for Candida albicans at the present time. This can contribute to immune system suppression or exhaustion.
- The symptoms of candidiasis often masquerade as symptoms of either allergy or hypoglycemia (low blood sugar). These three conditions, candidiasis, hypoglycemia and allergy often produce nearly identical symptoms. A person may have only one of these conditions at a time, or they may have all of them together at the same time. Those persons most severely ill with allergy usually have all three.

In summary, the points to remember are,

1. Allergic individuals frequently have Candida overgrowth.
2. Candida produces toxins that impair the immune system.
3. The Candida organism itself can be an allergen.
4. Candida can damage the intestinal lining, producing inflammation and promoting allergies.
5. Candida can migrate to many areas of the body and mutate into other forms.

Other Fungal Organisms

Although Candida is the most common of the fungal organisms in humans, there are other forms of fungi known to inhabit the human body. Often, these fungi gain a foothold in the body because of the already immunocompromised state brought about by Candida or other chronic infections. These other common fungi include:

Aspergillus

Aspergillus is a fungus that can reside in the lungs for years and cause asthma and breathing problems. This fungus that is commonly found in the environment growing on dead leaves, stored grain, bird droppings, compost piles, or other decaying vegetation. There are three ways that it causes illness in immunodeficient individuals.

1. Aspergillus is often involved in allergic reactions in people with asthma as it can colonize in a lung cavity and may produce a fungal ball called an aspergilloma.

2. Aspergillus may become an invasive infection with pneumonia and is then spread to other parts of the body through the blood stream. This invasive infection can affect and damage any organ of the body, especially the heart, lungs, brain, kidney, and eye.

3. Aspergillus can also appear in the sinuses leading to Aspergillus sinusitis with symptoms of stuffiness of the nose, chronic headache, or discomfort in the face.

Other symptoms of Aspergillus infection may include chest pain, cough, fever, joint pain, and a feeling of being "rundown."

Cryptococcus

Cryptococcosis is caused by a yeast-like organism, Cryptococcus neoformans, which is common in the environment, especially in soil containing bird excrement. Exposure occurs when these sources become airborne and are inhaled. Cryptococcosis is the most serious of the fungal infections in people with AIDS, usually manifesting as cryptococcal meningitis. Acute cryptococcal infection in almost every other organ of the body has also been described. Symptoms are very diverse and can be difficult to recognize. Fever, vomiting, headache, nausea, fatigue, loss of appetite, a general feeling of not being well are common symptoms as well as stiff neck and infrequently, seizures. Pneumonia may also be a sign of infection.

Histoplasma

Histoplasmosis is a fungal infection affecting the respiratory passages. It is thought to be acquired by breathing in the spores of the fungus found in soil contaminated by fecal droppings of birds and bats. The symptoms of histoplasmosis are acute shortness of breath,

81

coughing, fever, pains in the joints, ulcers of the gastrointestinal tract, spleen, liver enlargement, low white blood cell count, anemia, and adrenal necrosis. Histoplasmosis is not considered an allergic condition, but it can easily and frequently be mistaken for asthma.

Blastomyces

Blastomycosis is a fungal infection involving the lungs and occasionally spreading to the skin. When infection occurs in the lungs, it produces a dry, hacking cough sometimes with excess mucus. Chest pain, fever, chills, drenching sweats and shortness of breath are often initial symptoms. If untreated, the disease may slowly cause death.

More About Molds

Molds, which are inhaled, eaten or otherwise contacted, pack a double punch. Not only are they capable of producing substances that are toxic to the nerves and particularly to the central nervous system, but an individual may also be allergic to the specific mold. When both these conditions are present, the symptoms are magnified.

A characteristic of molds is that they produce antibiotics, which they release into the surrounding environment to kill competing bacteria in the vicinity. These fungal products are capable of damaging tissue cells, especially nerves. For example, the antibiotic cycloserine can cause hyperirritability, aggression, psychosis, drowsiness, and loss of memory, seizures, paralysis, convulsions and/or coma. These symptoms are clinically indistinguishable from the symptoms caused by psychic trauma.

Molds are known to produce symptoms three ways:

1. Molds give off toxins.
2. The immune system can produce antibodies, which lead to allergic reactions to a specific mold.
3. Molds cause an increase in the number and intensity of allergic reactions to foods and chemicals.

9

The Second Common Condition
Leading to Allergy: Parasites

Infestation of the human body by various forms of parasites is a condition that has not received the widespread attention it deserves. It is often unrecognized, undiagnosed and untreated by a majority of health professionals. This is in spite of the fact that the World Health Organization estimates that there are 1.2 billion people with roundworm, 1 billion with hookworm and 700 million with tapeworm, worldwide. Although many of these statistics reflect high levels of infestation in developing countries, it is becoming evident that parasitic infestation is far more common in North America than previously suspected. Regardless of the type of parasite that resides in the tissues, the end result of parasitic infection is toxicity, tissue damage and immune system suppression.

Apparently, one reason that parasites have been overlooked in North America is a general lack of formal training on the subject in most medical schools, coupled with a lack of information, and inadequate or unavailable diagnostic procedures. Nevertheless, clinical experience indicates that in people with allergy and related disorders, an estimated 80% respond favorably to an herbal parasite program.

Parasites are most likely to be present in immunocompromised individuals. People with parasitic disorders frequently have candidiasis or other fungal infections, which lower their immunity and make them more susceptible to parasitic infestation. Leo Galland, MD expressed this view in a 1988 issue of the *Townsend Letter for Doctors*. Dr. Galland wrote, "I strongly believe that every patient with disorders of immune function, including multiple allergies (especially food allergy) and patients with unexplained fatigue or with chronic bowel symptoms should be evaluated for the presence of intestinal parasites."

What is a Parasite?

A parasite is an organism that derives its food, nutrition and shelter by living in or on another organism and does not contribute beneficially to that organism. Many people, including many doctors think that only their pets or farm animals harbor parasites; or they assume that parasites are a disease found only in tropical countries. However, parasites show no socioeconomic boundaries and in fact they are found worldwide.

Dr. Hermann R. Bueno, Fellow of the Royal Society of Tropical Medicine and Hygiene of London, remarks, "Parasites are the missing diagnosis in the genesis of many chronic health problems, including diseases of the gastrointestinal tract and endocrine system. Most individuals would be truly amazed if they knew the extraordinarily high number of Americans who are unknowingly infected by parasites acquired during world travel or in the United States."

According to Ann Louise Gittleman in her book *Guess What Came To Dinner*, "Americans today are host to more than 130 different kinds of parasites, ranging from microscopic organisms to foot-long tapeworms."

Are there any indications that statistics like these hold true for Canada as well? In 1980 The National Research Council published *Intestinal Parasites in Man in the Canadian Environment* which states that there are 148 parasites in Canada; 64 of which are found in food and water. Between the years 1956 and 1978, Provincial Laboratories in British Columbia published a table of laboratory identifications of intestinal helminths (worms).

The most common types of worms identified in humans in this table are pinworm, whipworm, roundworm, and hookworm.

Pathogenic microorganisms have virulence factors and can cause disease in hosts with a normal defense capacity. Opportunistic microorganisms are considered those which cause disease only if the host resistance is sufficiently decreased. Parasitic infections are generally considered to be of the opportunistic variety.

How are Parasites Linked to Allergy?

Recent references in scientific literature suggest that parasites may be a primary cause of allergies. Although parasites in humans have been linked to allergic conditions for many years, today we have laboratory evidence of this link. It is known that parasites and their toxic waste products also stimulate the IgE antibody, which is usually involved in allergic responses with inhalants such as pollens and dust. Some tests also indicate that even after the parasitic infestation is brought under control, this IgE immune reaction may remain activated, turning its attention to other stimulants which initiates new allergies.

Many parasites can irritate and cause damage such as ulceration to the intestinal lining. This damage increases bowel permeability which then allows incompletely digested food particles to pass through to the bloodstream and initiate an allergic response, creating food allergies and intolerance. In one study, IgE antibodies were detected in 236 out of 312 food-sensitive people. In addition, increased levels of eosinophil s, a type of white blood cell often produced by parasitic infection, are characteristic. Eosinophils are associated with inflammation of the tissues, a typical picture in both allergic reactions and parasitic infestation.

Testing for Parasites

Testing for parasites has been notoriously inadequate for two reasons:
1. Most doctors are unaware of parasites in North America other than the highly publicized E. coli (Escherichia coli), Giardia, and cryptosporidium outbreaks. Therefore, most of their patients are not sent for testing.
2. Only a few laboratory tests for parasites exist. Dr. Ross Anderson estimates that, of the few individuals sent for testing, medical testing procedures catch only about 20% of the actual cases of parasites.

Dr. Zoltan Rona writes in his book *Childhood Illness and the Allergy Connection:*

The most accurate way of making a diagnosis of parasites is by what is known as a purged stool sample. Random stool analysis (not purged) will miss the diagnosis in over 50% of the cases. Many labs in the United States and Canada do not examine even purged stools with the appropriate stains or equipment.

Ann Louise Gittleman reports, "The traditional method for diagnosis of parasitic infestation...the search for cysts, trophozoites, ova, eggs, or worm segments in a random stool sample...is inaccurate and misleading for several reasons." These reasons are summarized in the following examples.

- Parasites such as filariasis, trichinosis and malaria reside in the tissue and blood and are not in the stool.
- Many parasites that do dwell in the gastrointestinal tract are known to strongly adhere to the intestinal mucosa and do not appear in the stools.
- The cyst, egg, or segment excretion rate can vary from day to day, requiring several stool samples to be taken on different days to make an accurate diagnosis.

Some of the tests that have been developed for parasites include the following.

Purged Stool Test

A purged stool test is good for identifying the presence of Giardia, amoebae, roundworm, threadworm, tapeworm, hookworm, cryptosporidium, liver flukes, blood flukes, strongyloides, and blastocystis. However, using this procedure, parasites rarely appear before the fourth evacuation and often as many as twelve bowel movements are required to yield a positive stool.

Rectal Swab

A small rectal speculum is used to obtain rectal mucus. This test has a high positive rate even when the purged sample is negative.

Blood Tests

When an elevated eosinophil (a type of white blood cell) count is found in a blood test, it is a strong indication of parasitic infection. Parasites that often cause an elevated eosinophil rate are roundworm, hookworm, toxocara, pinworms, and strongyloides. However, Giardia and amoebae rarely create eosinophilia.

Sputum Tests

Roundworm, hookworm, strongyloids, entamoeba histolytica, and Pneumocystis carinii have at times been found to produce positive sputum samples.

Urine Tests

Blood fluke eggs and microfilariae have been found in urine sediment.

Perineal Swabs

These swabs have revealed the presence of pork tapeworm, beef tapeworm, and blood fluke eggs. Transparent tape can be pressed against the anal and perineal areas and evaluated under a microscope to reveal the presence of pinworm.

Other Tests

Radiological tests, the String test, aspiration, biopsy, and cultures all can reveal specific types of organisms

Parasites damage the tissues in many ways. There is direct tissue damage in the area of the body they inhabit. Parasites feed on the body and the food of the human host, often creating nutritional deficiencies. They excrete waste products that are toxic and can damage tissues and place an increased demand on the immune system of the person infected.

Parasites are capable of creating nutritional deficiencies and imbalances. Some specific ways that parasites damage body tissues include the following.

1. They destroy cells in the body faster than the cells can be regenerated which may result in ulceration, perforation, or anemia. They also irritate the tissues, producing inflammatory reactions.
2. Parasites activate the immune system, which has the effect of overworking the system, eventually causing weakness and exhaustion of the immune system.
3. Parasites produce toxic waste products that harm the tissues of the body. This increase in toxic products must be neutralized by the body and may eventually lead to toxic overload.
4. Parasites produce a wide variety of symptoms because they can

inhabit any tissue of the body. Parasitic cysts have been found in the brain, spinal cord, eye, heart, and bones. These cysts can exert abnormal pressure on these organs. Other examples include pinworms that commonly inhabit the large intestine and appendix. Whipworm and threadworm are often found in the cecum, large intestine and ileum. Toxicara canis inhabits the liver, lungs, brain and eye. Filariasis is common to the lymphatics. Liver flukes are found in the bile ducts, lung flukes in the lungs. Fish tapeworm, beef tapeworm and pork tapeworm inhabit the small intestine. Toxoplasma gondii has been found in all the organs.

5. Parasites can create malnutrition through malabsorption of proteins, carbohydrates, fats, and especially vitamins A and B-12. In large numbers, parasites create iron deficiency anemia through blood loss. More study on this subject is urgently needed. It is known that roundworm and Giardia interfere with vitamin A absorption; hookworm can create iron deficiency anemia and B-12 loss is common with fish tapeworm infestation.

Parasites range in size from microscopic amoebae and protozoa to worms (like tapeworm) that can be several feet long. Every part of the body may be affected by either the parasite or its toxic waste products, producing many and diverse symptoms.

Common Symptoms of Parasitic Infestation

Abdominal cramps	Flu-like symptoms, coughing,
Anemia	sore throat, fever
Bloating	Food allergies and intolerance
Blood in stools	Grinding teeth at night
Brain fog	Impaired memory
Chest pains or heartburn	Inflammatory bowel disease
Chronic fatigue	Joint pain
Chronic, dry cough	Loss of appetite
Constipation	Muscle aches and pains
Diarrhea	Rash
Excessive appetite	Rectal itching
Excessive weight loss	Shortness of breath
Flatulence (excessive gas)	Sleep disturbances

How Parasites are Primarily Acquired

1. Ingestion in food, water, or other contaminated material
2. Skin contact with contaminated soil (for example, a hookworm burrowing into a bare foot)
3. Transplacentally (across the placental barrier) (for example, toxoplasmosis)
4. Through sexual activity
5. Injection of infective material (for example, a mosquito bite producing malaria)
6. Inhalation (for example, dust carrying parasitic cysts or spores)

Important Parasites in North America

The following parasites may be of concern to people in North America who have allergic symptoms or other unexplained chronic illness.

Nematodes (Roundworms) Ascaris lumbricoides

This large roundworm is the most common intestinal parasite in the world. It is estimated that 1.2 billion people are affected. Humans may be affected with many worms at one time since one female worm may release an average of 200,000 eggs per day. *Medical Parasitology* states, "The per capita worm burden may reach staggering levels, with hundreds or even thousands or more worms in a single individual." A Lancet editorial in 1989 stated that the Ascaris burden worldwide is so enormous that if placed head to tail the worms would encircle the globe 50 times.

This organism migrates out of the digestive tract into the blood and lymph, passing through various organs including the liver and lungs and creating tissue irritation and allergies. Occasionally the worms may migrate into the eyes, brain, and ears. In the intestines, roundworms consume large amounts of food and give off waste products, one of which is a foreign protein which causes the individual to have an allergic response.

Pinworm

The pinworm is the most common roundworm in the United

States and Canada. Pinworms are transmitted to humans through contaminated food, water, and human-to-human contact. These small worms inhabit various portions of the large and small intestine. The female crawls down the intestine and out of the anus to lay her eggs, which can number 5,000 to 16,000 eggs per day. Children are most commonly affected and itching around the anus is the most common pinworm symptom.

Hookworm

Hookworm is transmitted when the larvae, which inhabit warm, moist soil, penetrate the skin of the foot. It may also be transmitted by consuming contaminated fruits, vegetables, or water. The hookworm larvae travel through the bloodstream to the lungs, into the alveoli, then up the trachea, to the throat. From here they are swallowed and end up in the small intestine. They attach to the intestinal mucosa where they mature and consume large amounts of blood. When there is a considerable number of worms present in chronic infections, blood loss will be serious. The individual infected may become anemic and malnourished.

Whipworm

Whipworm is another common parasitic worm with worldwide distribution affecting an estimated 1 billion people. Humans become infected through the ingestion of eggs in contaminated soil, water, fruits or vegetables. One female may lay 3,000 to 7,000 eggs a day which develop in the small intestine and then travel to the large intestine. Here the worms inject a digestive fluid that converts the colon tissue into a liquid that the worms can consume. Light infections produce abdominal pain, tenderness, nausea, constipation, gas, slight fever and headaches. Heavier infections may result in bloody diarrhea, abdominal pain, weight loss, anemia and rectal prolapse.

Flukes

Flukes are flat leaf-shaped worms that grow up to 3.5 inches in length and can live up to thirty years in humans. The most common are liver flukes, lung flukes and intestinal flukes. Flukes are parasitic in nearly all of their life cycle forms and are very destructive to tissues. They are generally acquired by eating undercooked pork, fish, crab or infected water vegetation such as watercress, or water chestnuts. Also drinking, wading, or swimming in contaminated water may cause infection as the free-swimming larvae are able to penetrate the skin. Flukes possess two suckers that they use for attachment to their host. Flukes end up in various organs and release many eggs (up to 2400 eggs per day per worm) with tiny spines on the outside of them. As the eggs work their way to the digestive or urinary tract, the spines cause inflammation and tissue damage. These worms also release toxic waste products that may cause tissue damage. Flukes commonly inhabit the intestines, but they can also find their way to the liver, lungs, heart, brain, urinary bladder and blood vessels.

Liver Flukes

In humans, this fluke commonly inhabits the bile ducts of the liver and can create liver enlargement, liver abscesses or holes throughout the liver. Sometimes dead worms obstruct the common bile duct and occasionally flukes are found in the pancreatic duct where they can produce obstruction and acute pancreatitis. The worms may also invade the gallbladder. Long-standing infections may lead to the development of cancers. Fatigue is a common symptom of this fluke.

Lung Flukes

Eight different species of lung flukes are known to infect humans. Adult lung flukes are found in the lungs and even the brain where they have caused seizures similar to epilepsy. The immature parasite penetrates through the wall of the small intestine into the peritoneal cavity, and normally makes its way through the diaphragm and pleura into the lungs. Chronic infections may persist for many years. Symptoms may include a chronic mild cough and a bloodstained, brown, rusty-appearing sputum upon arising. Lung flukes can perforate lung tissue resulting in depleted oxygen supplies of the entire bloodstream. They weaken the lungs, which can lead to other illnesses and infections. On x-ray, the lungs will show signs similar to tuberculosis.

Intestinal Flukes

The adult intestinal fluke characteristically lives in the small intestine where it can cause ulceration. Other symptoms may include diarrhea, nausea, vomiting, abdominal pain and edema of the face. The parasite may migrate in the bloodstream to lodge inside weakened tissues such as the breast, lungs, and prostate. They can stimulate cancer cell division.

Blood Flukes

Blood flukes travel trough the bloodstream to several organs. They may attack the lining of the intestine, liver, bladder, urinary tract, or other pelvic organs. Symptoms may include a cough, arthritis-like symptoms, swollen lymph glands and diarrhea. They can also create blood clots. Some species of blood fluke release an enzyme that destroys the protein in the blood so they can consume the amino acids, especially arginine, causing a protein imbalance.

Protozoa

Protozoa are microscopic, single-celled organisms. This infection is usually transmitted in cyst form. The cysts are small, light, and easily ingested and human digestive juices do not destroy the cysts. They are capable of infecting every tissue in the body and they have an intensely rapid reproduction rate. Protozoa generally reproduce in the intestinal tract and then migrate to other organs and tissues or to the red blood cells. Individuals with weakened or stressed immune systems are particularly at risk. It is estimated that one fifth of the world's population is infected with Protozoa.

Diseases and Conditions Associated with Protozoal Infestation

Arthritis,	Multiple sclerosis.
Asthma	Ovarian cysts
Chronic fatigue	Psoriasis
Colitis	Swellings
Degenerative muscle diseases	Ulcers
Leukemia	Sores
Lymphoma	

Entamoeba Histolytica

This protozoan infects approximately 10% of the world's population. It principally inhabits the large intestine but may invade the mucosal crypts where it can feed on red blood cells and form ulcers. Damage can be extensive without showing clinical signs. Sometimes it will move through the capillaries to the blood stream and from there be carried to the liver, brain, lungs and heart and other organs where it can cause abscess formation. Massive food and environmental allergies have been reported with this infection.

Blastocystis Hominis

This organism was first considered a non-pathogenic yeast, but is now recognized by most researchers as a protozoan. Blastocystis Hominis is found in more stool specimens than any other parasite. Infection commonly occurs in the intestine at the site where the small intestine meets the colon. When present in large numbers, Blastocystis can suppress the immune system and cause gastrointestinal distress. This organism has been associated with allergies, headaches, nervous disorders, muscle aches, various forms of arthritis, irritable bowel disease and chronic fatigue.

Giardia

Giardia infects an estimated 18 million people. It has become better known than other parasites because of its contamination of much of the water supply in North America. It exists in both surface water and urban water systems. In 1965 there were several outbreaks in public water supplies which brought Giardia to the attention of the public. Since then, outbreaks have occurred intermittently in public water systems since chlorination does not always kill the cysts. Giardia apparently attaches itself to the walls of the upper intestine, inhibiting the body's ability to absorb nutrients.

The primary symptoms include sudden, explosive diarrhea, abdominal cramps, headaches, nausea, vomiting, and low-grade fever. The symptoms may vanish spontaneously, then come back again and again. Aside from an infected water supply, outbreaks have also been traced to contaminated food. Giardia is very contagious and day care centers may have a high incidence rate. Millions of Giardia cysts have been found in a just one soiled diaper. Immunocompromised individuals are especially at risk.

Cryptosporidium Parvum

The first two human cases of cryptosporidiosis were reported in 1976. Cryptosporidiosis is now recognized as a significant cause of diarrhea in humans and since 1984 it has been associated with outbreaks in child day care centers throughout the United States and Canada. A waterborne outbreak in Georgia in 1987 produced illness in an estimated 13,000 individuals. This was the first report of disease transmission by a municipal water system that was in compliance with all state and federal standards for water. Another outbreak in 1993 infected half the population of Milwaukee. The infective stage of this organism, the oocyst, is about half the size of a red blood cell. It has a rapid life cycle and huge numbers can colonize the small intestine in just a few days. Cryptosporidium may move to other locations in the intestines and in some immunocompromised individuals it has been found in the stomach, the ducts of the pancreas and liver and in the respiratory tract. It is spread by water or by eating contaminated food.

The main symptoms are diarrhea, abdominal cramps, weight loss and fever. In people with lung or trachea infections, coughing and low-grade fever are seen. Infections may be serious in immunocompromised individuals because of severe dehydration and electrolyte loss.

Tapeworms

Adult tapeworms inhabiting humans are the largest of the intestinal parasites. They have a flat and ribbon-like body, which consists of an attachment organ, or head, followed by a chain of segments. New segments grow throughout the life of the tapeworm. Except for the fish tapeworms, all tapeworms in humans have four muscular, cup-shaped suckers on the head. They inhabit the small intestine, where they attach to the mucosa and absorb nutrients, especially B-12 and folic acid, and give off toxic waste products.

These waste products may produce symptoms such as dizziness, unclear thinking, high or low blood sugar, hunger pains, poor digestion, and allergies.

Beef tapeworm has a worldwide distribution and is common in North America. Infection with beef tapeworm is acquired by eating rare or medium rare beef. In humans, beef tapeworm can reach several feet long and live up to 25 years. Usually, only one worm is present at a time in the intestine. The beef tapeworm usually does not produce marked symptoms other than abdominal discomfort, chronic indigestion, or diarrhea.

The pork tapeworm is acquired by eating raw or undercooked pork. It is a bit smaller than the beef tapeworm and multiple worms are usually present. Pork tapeworms cause the most damage to humans when the immature larvae invade the muscles, heart, eyes, or brain. This larval migration is the most dangerous infection of all the tapeworms.

The fish tapeworm is the largest of the human tapeworms, sometimes reaching up to 30 feet long. It is acquired by eating raw, undercooked, or pickled fish. A high prevalence of this parasite has been seen in Alaska and Canada. In the intestine, this parasite may consume 80% to 100% of the hosts' vitamin B-12, producing a condition similar to pernicious anemia. The individual may also experience pain and fullness in the upper abdomen, nausea, and anorexia.

All chronic parasitic infections tend to lead to allergic states in the body since they overwork the immune system. Parasites deplete nutrients and give off poisonous waste products that alter body functions. When lodged in a specific tissue, parasites often do direct damage to that tissue. It makes sense for anyone with allergies is to be checked thoroughly for parasites.

Negative Effects of Parasites
Malabsorption and nutrient depletion
Immunosuppression
Systemic allergic reactions

Herbal Treatment for Parasites
In general, herbal treatment for parasites is highly effective. Always sustain an herbal treatment for a minimum of 30 days. Parasites

have various cycles, going from eggs to larvae to mature forms, then laying more eggs. Some herbs work only on the adult parasite and therefore it is necessary to continue the herbs until all the cycles have been completed. Discontinuing too soon may allow eggs to hatch and the larvae to become established again. If in doubt, extend the length of time you take the herbs for another week or two.

Herbs Shown to be Effective in Treating Parasites

Black walnut is a traditional remedy for ringworm, athlete's foot and fungus as well as parasites and intestinal worms. It is the green outer hulls of the black walnut that are used. Black walnut is rich in organic iodine and tannins that have antiseptic properties.

Cloves are thought to kill the eggs of several types of parasites.

Garlic has several outstanding qualities. Over the years, garlic has been used for pinworms and other intestinal worms, but it also has antiviral, antibacterial and antifungal properties. The active part of garlic is allicin which is known to be effective against Entamoeba histolytica and Giardia lamblia.

Pumpkin seeds have been used as a folk remedy for tapeworms and roundworms.

Tansy is a traditional herb used to expel intestinal worms.

Wormwood (Artemisia annua) has been used for centuries for worms and parasites. One of its components is sesquiterpene lactone which works like peroxide and is believed to weaken parasite membranes. Tea of wormwood has been shown to be effective for pinworms and roundworms. Wormwood can kill adult and developmental stages of a broad spectrum of parasites.

Other remedies that have been shown to be effective for parasites include: barberry root bark, silverwood tea or juice, grapefruit seed extract, and proteolytic enzymes.

10

The Third Overlooked Condition Leading to Allergy: Digestive Difficulties

Digestion is too often taken for granted because it appears to proceed automatically without conscious awareness. People simply put food in their mouths and let the body do the rest. But is it really that simple? In fact, digestion is a very complicated process, nothing short of miraculous. Digestion is the cornerstone of good nutrition because without good digestion, nutrients cannot reach the cells to nourish the body. Furthermore, an incompetent digestive tract leads to allergies.

Twenty million Americans suffer from some form of indigestion, making it one of the most common ailments afflicting people today. Poor food choices, too much food, devitalized food, and processed, chemicalized food all have a negative impact on digestion. Various medications have been shown to damage the digestive tract.

In the United States, one out of three surgeries takes place because of digestive problems. One in ten deaths is attributed to digestive disorders. The vast majority of digestive conditions develop slowly over a long period of time. Many people think that if they do not have pain or discomfort in their stomachs, they do not have digestive disorders. They do not realize that excessive gas, belching, burning, bloating, heartburn, nausea, cramps, diarrhea and constipation are all symptoms signaling that the digestive process is not proceeding normally and should not be ignored.

Even worse, if you eat an average North American diet, you are virtually guaranteed to develop a chronic degenerative disease at some point in your lifetime. Of the top 10 major diseases which afflict an estimated 100 million Americans, 8 have been established as being diet-related and the other two have known dietary components. Diseases include: heart disease, obesity, alcoholism, cancer, diabetes, addiction, stroke, arthritis, mental illness and high blood pressure.

The Kellogg Report of May, 1990 by Joseph D. Beasley, MD and Jerry Swift, MA, explores the impact of nutrition, environment and lifestyle on the health of Americans:

Perhaps the clearest concrete example of the effects of nutritional inadequacy can be found in the elderly; one of the most basic reasons they catch pneumonia or break bones at far higher rates than others (and than they themselves did when younger) is that their resistance and resilience have long been undermined by inadequate nutrition. As we grow older we need fewer and fewer calories but just as many or more nutrients each day. Thus, we all require an increasingly nutrient-dense diet as the years pass, a need that is scarcely recognized and rarely met in contemporary America.

As our food supply is increasingly tampered with by all the various forms of processing, it is apparent that no race in history has ever attempted to live on the diet that North Americans are now eating. There is no scientific proof that we can healthfully live on it. There is considerable evidence that we cannot. More and more authorities are becoming aware that adequate diet is an absolutely necessary precondition to a healthy life.

Allergy can be characterized as a chronic degenerative disease which is diet-related, and is affecting more people today than ever before. Let's explore why.

Eating a diet high in fat, sugar and refined, processed foods alters normal digestion. While digestion may be the cornerstone of nutrition, it is also a cornerstone to understanding allergy. When you eat food, it goes through a series of chemical breakdowns called digestion. Proteins break down into amino acids, carbohydrates break down into glucose and fats break down into fatty acids. When this breaking down fails to happen, symptoms occur. When foods are fully digested, they enter the blood stream in the normal way. The body recognizes them as nutrients and utilizes them accordingly. If they are not in the correct form when they enter the blood stream, the body recognizes them as foreign invaders and attacks as if they were viruses or bacteria.

The most common food allergens are milk, egg, wheat, nuts, corn, soy and beef. All of these foods in various breakdown stages yield protein products. It is no coincidence that most food allergens are protein fragments from poorly digested meat, dairy products and the protein portion of wheat. Most bacteria and foreign invaders are also protein in nature, so the body is already programmed to attack unidentifiable protein particles. As noted previously, when food is fully digested into its proper end products, it has lost its ability to be allergenic.

Traditional medical treatment considers abstinence from the food allergen to be the most effective treatment. While this may relieve symptoms, it will not get the person well. Avoiding the food is treating the symptom rather than the cause. The egg is not the cause of the patient's symptoms, although the egg may very well induce all kinds of reactions. Helping an incompetent digestive tract to work better is a more rational approach. It is necessary to eliminate the egg only until the digestive tract is healed and functioning normally. If you can't digest the egg, you can't get its nutrients, but you can get allergic reactions.

Amino acids are the end products of protein digestion. It is the amino acid which is absorbed from the intestine and circulated in the blood to the cells. The cells are extremely creative with these amino acids. They link them together in chain-like structures, to make new proteins capable of specific functions. Each cell is a mixture of proteins and a single cell can contain hundreds of combinations of proteins.

For example in the lottery game 6/49, six numbers are picked from a possible 49 numbers. We are told there are approximately 14 million combinations possible from these 49 numbers. We know that there are about 20 major amino acids in the body and thousands of lesser-known amino acids. Even with just the 20 amino acids, we have the possibility of more than seven million combinations if they were linked six at a time. However, the average number of amino acids linked together in the body is 400 and even the smallest protein has 20 amino acids, not six. The actual number of combinations possible is estimated to be infinite. Because of these infinite possibilities, it doesn't make sense to try to control each little step in the digestive process.

The control you have is with the lifestyle choices you make as to what you eat, drink, think and expose your body to. Having a better understanding of digestion and what your digestive needs are will help you to make more appropriate choices. It also gives you an opportunity to prevent digestive problems from arising.

The Digestive Process

Digestion begins in the mouth where two processes act to break down the food. Chewing breaks up large chunks of food while saliva coats the food and allows the enzymes contained in the saliva to begin their work. After swallowing, it takes about six seconds for the food to move through the esophagus to the stomach. Here the saliva enzymes may continue their digestive activity because, although they work in an alkaline environment, it will take the stomach 45 minutes to an hour to secrete sufficient hydrochloric acid to neutralize the saliva enzymes.

Enzyme activity is dependent upon the pH of the fluid that surrounds the enzymes. Each enzyme works within a very specific pH range. The enzymes from the saliva work in an alkaline solution, and hence are inactivated in an acid stomach environment. However, other enzymes now go to work.

Where does hydrochloric acid come from?

Basically, it comes from the blood. When food enters the stomach, the stretching of the stomach lining signals the parietal cells along the stomach's mucous membrane to begin secreting hydrochloric acid. In order to do this, the cells must pull hydrogen and chloride ions from the blood. These pass through the parietal cells and

100

are combined in the stomach to become hydrochloric acid. Hydrochloric acid does not digest food. It stimulates an inactive enzyme called pepsinogen to become active. This active form, called pepsin, begins splitting protein particles into smaller fragments. The stomach lining is protected from its highly acid contents by a thick layer of mucus. Food stays in the stomach two to four hours, depending on the types of foods eaten.

The acid chyme is now slowly passed or squeezed through the pyloric valve into the small intestine. The small intestine is not really small; it is 15 to 20 feet long and it has been said that if it were spread flat, that it would cover a surface area the size of a tennis court. This is a huge absorptive surface for nutrients to pass through. The intestinal lining has the capacity to repair and replace itself every 3 to 5 days. The highly acid food entering the small intestine encounters an alkaline environment, created by bicarbonate secreted in large amounts by the pancreas. The acid stomach enzymes are now inactivated by the alkalinity of the small intestine, but the pancreas will now additional enzymes to work in this final digestive process. Protein, carbohydrate and fat-digesting enzymes are all supplied on demand by the pancreas.

Bile

The gallbladder stores and concentrates bile that has been produced by the liver. Bile contributes some interesting functions to the digestive process. Oils and fats must first be emulsified by bile (which contains no digestive enzymes) in order for digestive enzymes to penetrate them. If bile is too thick or the supply of bile is insufficient, digestion is severely restricted. Food will be incompletely digested and may accumulate in the lower digestive tract where putrefaction can take place. Insufficient hydrochloric acid production is always associated with poor bile flow.

Certain foods stimulate bile flow more than others do. Protein has a strong stimulus on bile flow with carbohydrates slightly less. Cabbage, cucumbers, radishes, onions and apples strongly stimulate bile flow. Paradoxically, while fats require bile before they can be digested, fats are not a strong stimulus for the flow of bile. When bile is not flowing adequately, gas, bloating and abdominal discomfort may result. Other symptoms include constipation and light-colored stools, sour taste in the mouth, loss of appetite especially for meat, and gallbladder stones.

What Happens when Things Go Wrong with Digestion?

Abnormal digestion may not necessarily produce pain, so a person may not know when digestion is no longer competent. If pain is produced, however, it is a major warning flag. If a person seeks medical help at this time, often no tissue changes have taken place that can be diagnosed as a disease. After months or years of incompetent digestion and ever-increasing symptomatology, recognizable tissue changes may result, and the diagnosis of disease is finally made.

Somewhere in between, allergies often develop, because any time there is tissue injury in the digestive tract, large, undigested food particles have the opportunity to enter the blood stream. The resultant attack on these food particles by the immune system creates the allergic reaction.

Health professionals have long noted that the symptoms of too much stomach acid as well as too little stomach acid can be strikingly similar. Both conditions can produce symptoms of burping, bloating, upset stomach, burning, gas, and a sense of fullness following meals.

Too Much Acid

Most people with stomach symptoms assume that they have too much hydrochloric acid. They look for ways to neutralize this acid rather than trying to determine why or even if the acid is there in the first place. A main cause of over acidity is overfilling the stomach (eating too much). This stretches the stomach lining which, as we have seen, is the stimulus for the cells to secrete hydrochloric acid. Similarly, fried or fatty foods cause the food to stay in the stomach for a longer period of time, stimulating acid build up.

Symptoms are not caused by a particularly low (very acid) pH of the secretions, but rather by abnormally large amounts of gastric secretion in the stomach. Poor eating habits such as eating too fast and not chewing the food well may overstimulate the acid producing glands. Anxiety and stress is thought to play a role. Heartburn can be caused by reflux of the acid stomach contents into the bottom part of the esophagus which occurs when the esophageal sphincter muscle is relaxed. Foods that may relax the sphincter muscle are fats, alcohol, chocolate and coffee.

What Happens when Antacids are Used?

Antacids alkalinize the only organ in the body that is supposed to be acid. They control secretions of hydrochloric acid by turning off all digestion in the stomach and thereby putting the entire stress of digestion on the pancreas.

Antacids disrupt the blood stream as well as the stomach with alkalinity. This makes the hydrogen in the blood unavailable to the parietal cells to form hydrochloric acid because the blood must maintain a narrow pH range and the removal of hydrogen ions would create further alkalinity in the blood. If hydrochloric acid cannot be formed, the stomach enzymes cannot work, as they require an acid pH of around 2 to 3. Since pepsin works on protein, protein digestion in the stomach cannot take place efficiently. This has the effect of increasing the number of partially digested, large protein molecules entering the systemic circulation as well as the lower bowel. Chronic use of antacids causing decreased stomach acidity can also impair the absorption of minerals.

Too Little Acid

Medical studies reveal that too little stomach acid is found in 14% to 20% of patients in the hospital for conditions other than gastric conditions. There is also evidence that between 25% to 35% of patients over 60 years of age produce too little acid. Without adequate acid levels, the body has a hard time digesting food, particularly proteins. When not properly digested, proteins putrefy in the intestines and bacteria acts on them to produce foul-smelling gas. Without sufficient acid, the pancreas is not stimulated to release pancreatic enzymes into the small intestine, severely compromising the digestion and absorption of all food categories and vitamins A and E and B-12. The assimilation of many minerals, including calcium is dependent on an adequate supply of hydrochloric acid. Hydrochloric acid is also necessary to keep bacteria that live in the colon from translocating up into the small intestine. Undesirable strains of bacteria and yeast can take hold and multiply in portions of the intestine where they are not normally found, further interfering with digestion and absorption. These bacteria and yeasts may also irritate and inflame the intestines, creating hyperpermeability and initiating food reactions.

Disorders associated with too little stomach acid include; asthma, celiac disease, chronic autoimmune disorders, eczema, food allergies and intolerance, gall bladder disease, psoriasis, acne, chronic hives, undigested food in stool, chronic Candida infections, and osteoporosis.

Dr. James Braly estimates that 80% or more of food-allergy sufferers have differing degrees of low stomach acid leading to poor digestion and creating the numerous spin-off problems previously mentioned.

The vital function of digestion is primarily dependent upon the pH of the blood, and the pH of the blood is dependent to a large degree upon the food that is eaten. The reason that digestion is dependent upon the pH of the blood is that the acid-forming elements, hydrogen and chloride, must be present in the blood in sufficient quantities for the stomach's parietal cells to place the end product of hydrochloric acid in the stomach. Parietal cells communicate with the blood through a system of intracellular caniculi. If the blood has too much alkalinity, hydrochloric acid formation in the stomach is diminished, because the blood will not release its acid substances.

The Small Intestine

A similar situation occurs in the small intestine. When the acidic stomach contents enter the small intestine, the pH of the small intestine falls below 4.0, which is acid. However, digestion here requires an alkaline pH. The acidity triggers an enzyme called secretin to be released in large quantities, stimulating the immediate release of bicarbonate which is very alkaline. The alkaline bicarbonate is formed in the ductile cells of the pancreas from substances extracted from the blood. If the concentration of these substances is below their respective thresholds, they will remain in the blood and not be available for the purpose of digestion. This is because maintenance of blood pH gets first priority for survival. Only when a sufficient quantity of materials is present in the blood can they be released for digestive purposes.

How do Drugs Interfere With the Intricate Digestive Process?

Over-the-counter and prescription drugs can exert many adverse effects on the intestine and its processes. Non-steroidal anti-inflammatory drugs (NSAIDS), aspirin, and steroids such as prednisone and cortisone can suppress repair of the intestine. They have also been shown to increase gut permeability. Long-term steroid use may cause stomach and duodenal ulcers which contribute significantly to intestinal hyperpermeability.

Antibiotics disrupt the normal balance of bacterial microflora in the gut which can lead to overgrowth of pathogenic organisms. Infection and inflammation may result as well as the loss of some vitamins produced by the friendly intestinal bacteria. Symptoms of gas, bloating, and gastrointestinal distress further interfere with the digestive process.

Your Intestinal Microflora

The colon microflora is often called the "garden within." How we cultivate this garden can mean the difference between radiant health and chronic debilitating conditions. The adult human intestine contains approximately 3.5-4.5 lbs. of microorganisms. More than 500 different species of organisms are normally present in a healthy person as well as some potentially harmful organisms (pathogens). Few people realize that this vast colony of microflora is necessary for health and prevention of disease. In fact, some authorities estimate that the intestine makes up to 80% of the immune system. According to the book *Human Intestinal Flora*, Drasar & Hill, 1974, "The intestine is one of the major sites of immunological activity." This resource further states that "The metabolic activity of the gut flora is potentially equal to that of the liver". These normal microorganisms participate in many functions important to the health of the body.

The type and quantity of these beneficial organisms are directly affected by the diet. The food eaten is also food for the bacteria. The more a certain type of food is eaten, the more the bacteria specific to it can grow. For example, when a high protein diet is eaten, proteolytic bacteria proliferate in the intestine.

In a healthy colon, the friendly bacteria hold pathogens in check. Balance or imbalance of these organisms has far-reaching effects on the quality of one's health. This natural microflora of the bowel, a vast colony of organisms within the body, is necessary for life, health, and the prevention of disease. These bacteria live in a symbiotic role which means that both the person and the bacteria mutually benefit from each other. When the optimal balance between friendly and unfriendly organisms is adversely altered by disruptive factors in our external or internal environments, the resulting unhealthy condition is called dysbiosis.

Main Causes of Dysbiosis

1 Antibiotics, antacids, steroid drugs such as cortisone and birth control pills, and non-steroidal, anti-inflammatory drugs (NSAIDS). Familiar names for NSAIDS are: aspirin, Ibuprofen, Motrin, Advil, Aleve, Nanaprox, Feldene, Flexeril, Indocin, Naprosyn, Ketoprofen.
2 Poor or imbalanced diet, too much sugar.
3 Poor digestion of food and/or poor elimination of wastes.
4 Chlorinated water when used on a regular basis.
5 On-going negative stress.
6 Radiation (X-rays).

What Are the Functions of Your Friendly Bacteria?

In the last ten years, more information has become available on the intestinal flora and their contributions to health than ever before. Understanding the many vital protective functions these bacteria perform helps them attain their proper place of importance.

Some of the most common of the friendly bacteria include L. acidophilus, L. bulgaris, L casei, L. bifidus, L. salivarius, streptococcus lactis and streptococcus thermophilus.

Friendly Bacteria

- Manufacture B vitamins such as biotin, niacin (B-3), pyridoxine (B-6), folic acid, pantothenic acid and vitamin B-12.
- Have powerful anti-tumor potentials (anti-carcinogenic)
- Help to control unhealthy organisms by altering the acidity of the region they inhabit. Some produce specific antibiotic substances and other protective products -antibacterial, antifungal, and antiviral. They deprive some undesirable organisms of their nutrients.
- Help to control cholesterol levels by digesting fats into healthy fatty acids.
- Enhance immune system function by protecting against the negative effects of radiation and pollutants.
- Enhance and help normalize bowel function.
- Aid digestion by helping the digestive system to break down food into simpler, more usable forms that can then be absorbed by the body.
- Aid in the overall efficiency of digestion, absorption and assimilation of nutrients.
- Produce butyric acid by feeding on vegetable fiber. Butyric acid helps nourish the lining of the colon.
- Make short-chain fatty acids from carbohydrates that supply both the intestinal tract and the body with energy. Short-chain fatty acids are also essential for maintaining healthy intestinal barrier functions.
- Protect against parasites by keeping some parasites from transforming into more aggressive, disease-causing strains.
- Help maintain an optimal intestinal lining which protects against irritating allergy-causing substances.
- Produce some digestive enzymes.
- Detoxify bile in the intestinal tract and deactivate many toxic pollutants.
- Help keep the pH (acid-alkaline balance) of the intestine optimal. This optimizes digestion and further protects against disease-causing organisms that tend to grow in an abnormally altered pH.
- Appear to play a role to increase the absorption of minerals such as calcium, magnesium, and in some cases, iron.
- Aid digestive disorders such as indigestion, belching, gas, constipation and diarrhea.

What Symptoms are Linked to Improper Bowel Flora?

When the bowel ecology is not in optimum condition, important immune functions and protection is lost and symptoms begin to emerge. Some of the symptoms linked to improper bowel flora include:

Acne	Hormonal disturbances
Arthritis	Intestinal symptoms
Asthma	Irregular heartbeat
Ear inflammation	Low back pain
Fatigue	Nervousness
Headaches	Rashes

Probiotics

When the intestinal flora has been disrupted, probiotics can help to replace the lost organisms and aid the intestine to regain a healthful balance. Probiotics, meaning, pro life are live beneficial bacteria in supplement form. Since they are alive, heat, light, and moisture can adversely affect these organisms. A good guideline for probiotics is that they should be refrigerated both in the store where you buy them and when stored in your home.

Recommended therapeutic dose of probiotics is around 18 to 20 billion organisms per day. and about 3 to 7 billion organisms per as a maintenance dose.

The strain of the type of bacteria can be important. It must be able to survive the stomach digestive acids and the bile acids, attach itself to the intestinal wall and be acceptable to the immune system. Some L. acidophilus strains which are known to perform these functions are INT 9, DDS-1 and NAS strains.

For healing purposes, the powdered form is preferable, as it is an easy way to consume the required larger dose. However, capsules are also acceptable.

Fiber Facts

Insufficient fiber contributes to 29% of digestive disorders. Fiber helps to prevent and heal a variety of gastrointestinal problems such as ulcers, irritable bowel syndrome, inflammatory bowel disease, and hemorrhoids. A 1984 article in the *British Journal of Nutrition* claims that fiber reduces hunger and beneficially influences carbohydrate and fat metabolism. Fiber is a must for keeping the bowel healthy.

There are two classes of dietary fiber:

1. Insoluble fiber is found in grains, vegetables, and most bran. This fiber produces the bulk of the stool and helps to maintain healthy stool transit time. This fiber has been characterized as an intestinal broom which sweeps sticky food and other waste from the bowel wall. It also absorbs toxins. Insoluble fiber holds three times its weight in water.

2. Soluble fiber is found in fruits and some vegetables. Other examples are psyllium, legumes, beans and oats. Soluble fiber holds more than fifty times its weight in water and also has wide-ranging positive effects on intestinal function. This fiber helps maintain healthy levels of friendly bacteria. Pectin found in apples and citrus fruits resist digestion and absorption but bind to substances such as cholesterol and heavy toxic metals. They are known to protect the colon against cancer. Pectin holds one hundred times their weight in water.

The National Cancer Institute recommends eating an average of 25 grams of fiber a day. Most people eat only about half that amount, 12 grams of fiber per day. A study at McMaster University demonstrated that a diet including 30 grams of insoluble fiber daily would significantly decrease the cholesterol level in the blood.

Another important consideration for health is the length of time it takes for food to travel through the intestines. This is called the transit time and an ideal transit time is considered to be 12 to 18 hours. The longer the transit time, the greater the possibility that putrefaction of food may occur and yield unhealthy waste products which can be absorbed into general circulation. A major determining factor in reducing transit time is the addition of fiber to the diet.

Transit time can be checked at home by swallowing a few whole kernels of corn or a half dozen charcoal capsules. Time how long it takes for these products to show up in the stool.

Bowel Toxins

Numerous toxins are produced in the colon, especially where there is alteration of the ratio of normal flora to pathogenic flora. Increased numbers of pathogenic organisms can produce pathogenic substances. For example, Candida and other yeasts ferment dietary sugars to ethyl alcohol and acetylaldehyde. They also increase the permeability of the intestine, allowing their toxic products to enter the blood stream.

Many toxic products of bacterial decomposition are known to be absorbed from the intestine into the blood stream. These products are conveyed to the liver for detoxification. The fact that toxins are absorbed from the intestine is evidenced in many laboratory studies. However, some toxins may be present in too large a quantity for the liver to detoxify, or there may be toxins produced that the liver cannot detoxify.

Indole is formed from tryptophan, an amino acid derived from protein and delivered to the liver for detoxification. This is the basis for the common urine indican test as a measure of protein digestion. Indole gives a characteristic foul odor to feces.

Phenol is an example of a toxin produced in the bowel from the amino acid tyrosine in the process of putrefaction. Phenol is toxic to the body and irritates tissues as it circulates through the blood. Unfortunately, the liver cannot detoxify phenol. Phenol has the ability to kill cells, especially liver and kidney cells. The presence in the blood of toxic products of decomposition can be increased by any defect of the intestinal lining.

Ammonia is another substance produced in the intestine by bacterial action on proteins. If ammonia enters the blood stream, neurological symptoms may develop, such as confusion, drowsiness, mental disturbances, tremors and altered EEG patterns. Ammonia is normally converted in the liver to urea. However, when the amount of ammonia overwhelms the liver's capacity to convert the ammonia, neurological symptoms have been observed.

Many toxins produced by microflora have not been studied in great detail, but the few that have been studied should alert us to the importance of maintaining healthy flora in the intestines.

Diet Producing the Lowest Levels of Toxins

(most efficient in lowering toxin production and increasing nutrient values)

1. A low protein, high complex carbohydrate diet with abundant fresh fruits and vegetables.
2. A diet in which small to moderate amounts of food are eaten. All food, if eaten in too great a quantity for the digestive enzymes to process, can lead to the production of toxins.

11

Enzymes: The Rescue Remedy

Enzymes are proteins (in the form of amino-acid chains) secreted by cells and found in every cell of the body. They control the rate of reactions and responses that direct, accelerate, retard or modify all cell functions to supply energy and nutrients. Technically, enzymes act to induce chemical changes in other substances without undergoing change themselves. Although originally thought not to be used up during reactions, evidence is emerging that enzymes eventually do wear out and are discarded by the body. An enzyme is composed of two parts; a protein part and a cofactor (often a vitamin or mineral).

Scientists consider enzymes to be organic compounds capable of accelerating or producing some change in (by breaking down) a substance for which they are usually specific. However, Dr. Howell describes enzymes as specialized "protein carriers charged with vital energy factors." He likens them to the battery of a flashlight. When the battery has energy, the flashlight lights up. When the battery is dead, it will not activate the flashlight. However, the battery itself looks the same in both cases. Dr. Howell believes enzymes work the same way. An example is two seeds. The first seed is planted in the soil. The second seed is boiled first and then planted. Only the first seed will grow because it contains live enzymes, although both seeds look the same. The growing seed is an example of enzyme activity. Other examples of enzyme activity are ripening of fruit and leaves changing color in the fall. In the human body, absolutely every activity requires enzymes: eating, breathing, sleeping, working and even thinking. Metabolism is involved in all these activities and enzymes are what keeps the metabolism working.

The amino acids derived from protein have long been considered to be the building blocks of the cell. However, the enzymes are the workers that put the amino acids together. This is the difference between having a pile of bricks and having a brick house. The bricks (amino acids) cannot be put together without workers (enzymes). Every activity of the body is dependent upon enzymes. Enzymes digest food, activate the immune system and build minerals into bone. Male sperm carries enzymes that dissolve part of the female egg membrane in order for the sperm to gain entrance to the ovum and fertilize it.

Each organ and tissue has its own specialized enzymes to do the work required. Ninety-eight different enzymes have been found in the arteries alone, helping to keep them clean and functional. In fact, a whole book on just the enzymes in the arteries has been written. About 5,000 individual enzymes have so far been isolated and identified, but some authorities estimate that it takes about 100,000 enzymes to run the body, each with a specific job to do.

Is It Possible to Have an Enzyme Deficiency?

The answer is yes and that is why it is important to know about enzymes. Some enzyme deficiencies are well documented, such as lactase deficiency. When this enzyme is deficient, a person can experience gas, bloating, diarrhea, gastritis and pain from drinking milk simply because that one enzyme is lacking. When the enzyme phenylalanine hydroxylase is absent in babies, phenylalanine accumulates in the tissues and can kill or mentally retard the baby unless it is treated. This condition is called phenylketonuria or PKU. Dr. Jonathan Brostoff reports on an experiment done on chemical and food sensitive individuals in *The Complete Guide to Food Allergy and Intolerance.* In the group which was sensitive to chemicals, 90% were deficient for one enzyme. In the food intolerant group, 80% were deficient for one enzyme.

What Are the Symptoms of Enzyme Deficiency?

Enzyme deficiency is characterized by producing insidious, chronic degenerative and chronic inflammatory changes. Redness, swelling, pain, abnormal motion, disturbed digestion and chronic illness are frequent signs of enzyme deficiency. Gradually, scientists are becoming aware that the digestive organs that produce digestive enzymes are not large enough to produce all the enzymes needed when enzyme deficient, processed and packaged foods predominate in the diet. When the body is burdened with an accumulation of food that it cannot efficiently digest and assimilate, food allergies and intolerance, gas, bloating, heartburn, constipation and diarrhea are some of the symptoms that may be produced. However, these symptoms may result over time in producing more serious metabolic changes.

The body's ability to function, repair injured tissues and ward off disease is directly related to the strength and numbers of its' enzymes. Disease, enzyme deficient foods, stress, physical injuries, aging and digestive problems can all affect tissue enzyme levels. Inadequate digestive enzyme activity is related to chronic inflammations, recurrent infections, and inability to gain or lose weight.

Enzyme Inhibitors

Besides deficiency, some substances are enzyme inhibitors that actually inhibit the activity of enzymes. Most medications including aspirin are examples of enzyme inhibitors. Organic solvents produced from petroleum or natural gas are used in many manufacturing processes and are known to inhibit a wide variety of enzymes. Organic solvents include methanol, ethanol, propenol, formic acid, ethylene glycol, hexane, benzene and butanol. These chemicals can be found in numerous everyday products including paints and household cleaners.

Some foods contain enzyme inhibitors. Seeds, nuts, grains, and beans contain enzyme inhibitors which should be deactivated prior to eating by soaking, cooking, or sprouting. Soaking or sprouting results in replacing enzyme inhibitors with abundant energizing enzymes.

Is it Too Simple?

Understanding the basic need of the body to be able to digest what it eats is a point that is all too often glossed over by health professionals. It is often just assumed that if it is eaten, the body will digest it even though indigestion is one of the most prevalent health problem today. Although it is a well-accepted fact that proper nutrition is vital to the maintenance of a healthy body, the actual way that the body achieves optimum nutrition is too often overlooked. Rarely is a person's ABILITY TO DIGEST FOOD evaluated as a possible cause for nutritional deficiencies and subsequent ill health. This is in spite of the fact that proper digestion of food is a preliminary step in the effective absorption and utilization of nutrients by the body. Instead, nutritional deficiencies are simply assumed to be the result of inadequate intake of nutrients.

Three categories of enzymes are of particular importance to health; Digestive enzymes that digest food, metabolic enzymes that run the body and food enzymes that are found in raw food.

Digestive enzymes

Digestive enzymes are the enzymes that are produced by the body to digest food when it is eaten. Secreted by glands, they are found in saliva, stomach and small intestine fluids and pancreatic juice. Their role is to break down food into small enough particles that they can be absorbed through the intestine and be utilized as nutrients.

Metabolic enzymes

These enzymes are produced by the body and perform various complex biochemical reactions within the tissues, including the activities of the immune system.

Food Enzymes

Raw foods in their natural state contain enzymes that, when activated, help to digest the food. When these raw foods are eaten, the enzymes in the food are activated and begin the process of digestion, which can significantly contribute to the complete digestion of the food.

Enzymes Have Special Needs.

Enzymes have very specific environmental needs in order to become active and work. These needs are specific pH range, specific temperature range, specific substrate (substance to work on) and moisture.

pH

Each type of enzyme has its specific acid/alkaline range(pH) in which it works . The enzyme chymotrypsin can only work in a very alkaline range, while pepsin must have a very acid environment. If pepsin is put in an alkaline solution, it is inactivated.

Temperature

Enzymes also have their own particular temperature range. They are inactive outside that range. A pear will ripen at room temperature faster than a pear put in the refrigerator, because the pear at room temperature will have more enzyme activity.

Substrate

Each enzyme works only on a specific substance. For example, the enzyme lipase will break down fat, not protein or carbohydrate. Protease can only digest protein; it cannot break down carbohydrate or fat.

Moisture

Most enzymes require moisture to become active. Enzymes stored in a dry form such as in a supplemental capsule remain inactive for months until they are swallowed. They are activated as soon as they are mixed with body fluids.

Chewing Helps Food Allergy

Enzymes are the keys to eliminating allergy. It has been said that 90% of all food allergy could be eliminated if people chewed their food well. When food is chewed well, it is thoroughly mixed with enzymes from the saliva. Enzymes work on the surfaces of the food particles which means that the more thoroughly chewed the food is, the more exposed surfaces there are for enzymes to work on. In fact, studies done at the University of Illinois have demonstrated that up to 80% of the carbohydrates can be digested by saliva enzymes alone. Also, the cells of fruits and vegetables have an indigestible cellulose layer which must be broken down by chewing before the fruit or vegetable can be digested. Many adverse reactions to fresh produce result simply from not chewing sufficiently to break down the cellulose membranes to allow the enzymes contained within the cells to work.

The teeth are very efficient if allowed to do their work. Using the jaw muscles, studies show that the front teeth (incisors) can close with a force of up to 55 pounds. The back teeth (molars) can close with a force of up to 200 pounds. With a small piece of food between the molars, the actual force per square inch can be up to several thousand pounds.

Enzyme Depleters

Cooking food depletes enzymes. When food is heated above 118° F, virtually all of the enzymes naturally occurring in the food are destroyed. In addition, cooking food can either destroy or make unavailable up to 85% of the original nutrients.

Other food preparation methods that deplete enzymes are milling and refining, commercial drying, canning, commercial freezing, and irradiation. Chemicals added to food in the form of preservatives, coloring agents, synthetic flavors and flavor enhancers, and pesticides all tend to inhibit enzyme activity.

Enzyme Helpers

What are the foods that contain a high content of enzymes? Raw meat and unpasteurized milk products are high in enzyme content. Today, however, these uncooked foods are either unsafe or unavailable and cannot be recommended. Fresh fruits and vegetables are excellent sources of enzymes, although the enzyme density is not as high in these high water products. Juicing raw fruits and vegetables tends to concentrate the enzymes and allows increased enzyme intake as well as easy absorption of nutrients. Fermented foods are generally high in enzyme content which is one reason that they are easy to digest. Fermented foods include yogurt, kefir, sauerkraut, soy sauce, miso, tempeh, and kimchi and quality cheese. Lactic acid bacteria used to ferment some of the above foods contain proteolytic enzymes and lactose-digesting enzymes. The finished product is higher in enzyme content than the original material.

Yogurt is fermented milk with enhanced digestibility because of its composition of living microorganisms. Quality yogurt contains live and active cultures. If these living cultures have been destroyed which is the case with many pasteurized supermarket brands, the product can no longer be considered a true yogurt and its primary health benefits have been lost.

118

Kefir, a fermented milk product used for thousands of years as a traditional food in many parts of the world, is considered to be one of the richest sources of enzymes. Kefir is easier to digest than yogurt and milk used to make kefir does not have to be preheated like milk used for making yogurt.

Homemade sauerkraut contains active enzymes. The enzymes have been destroyed in some commercial sauerkraut, especially canned.

Tempeh is fermented soybeans and kimchi is Korean pickled vegetables.

Raw honey is another enzyme dense product. Enzymes are important in the honey ripening process, in the flavor and color of honey and are partly responsible for honeys' antiseptic and healing properties.

Sprouted seeds, beans, grains, and nuts are enzyme-rich. Enzyme activity is increased through the sprouting process. For example, when wheat is sprouted, the protease activity increases 15 times.

Types of Enzymes

Under normal circumstances, the body is capable of producing the following enzymes: protease, lipase, amylase and disaccharidase. The body does not produce cellulase

Protease

Protease breaks down (hydrolyzes) proteins into amino acids. Foods that contain high levels of protease (before cooking) include meats, eggs, milk, and natural cheese. Soy, wheat, barley, bulgur, wild rice and peanuts also contain high levels. In addition to digesting proteins in foods, protease can digest microorganisms composed of protein such as the protein coating on some viruses and bacteria.

A protease deficiency compromises the immune system which can result in chronic infections, chronic inflammations, fluid retention and fluid in the ears. Protease has been shown to be absorbed through the intestine in substantial quantities where it enters the bloodstream and binds to serum proteins. Tissues involved with immune function can then utilize it.

Calcium is carried in the blood partly bound to digested protein. Inadequate protein digestion can lead to calcium utilization problems which include osteoporosis, osteoarthritis, degenerative disc problems and bone spurs.

Lipase

Lipase breaks down (hydrolyzes) fats into monoglycerides and fatty acids. Foods that contain high levels of lipase include raw seeds, nuts, bananas, cherries, figs and grapes. Lipase is important to maintain optimum cell permeability so that nutrients can easily flow into the cell and waste materials can flow out. Lack of lipase can cause interference with insulin metabolism and the transport of glucose into the cell by insulin. Lipase deficiency may also result in a tendency towards high cholesterol and high blood triglycerides, high blood pressure, difficulty losing weight and varicose veins.

Amylase

Amylase breaks down (hydrolyzes) carbohydrates into simple sugars and glucose. High levels of amylase are found in fruits and grains. Amylase possesses antihistamine properties and is helpful in skin problems such as hives and rashes, eczema and allergic reactions to bee stings, and bug bites. Amylase combined with certain herbs has been shown to alleviate the wheezing of asthmatics,

Disaccharidase

Disaccharidases digest simple sugars found in dairy products, grains, and white sugar and flour. The three major disaccharides are sucrose (table sugar), lactose (milk sugar) and maltose (grain sugar). Eating too much sugar may compromise the body's ability to produce enough disaccharidases to keep up with the demand. When not enough enzyme is present for the amount of sugar intake, sugar intolerance can develop. Deficiency of disaccharidases is a very common source of intestinal discomfort, gas and bloating.

Disaccharidases are located in the microvilli of the intestine. Certain diseases such as gluten intolerance can damage these microvilli and seriously impair the activity of their disaccharidases. In fact, these very important enzymes are subject to damage from several sources. For example, folic acid and/or B-12 deficiency may prevent proper development of the microvilli. Too thick a layer of mucus can inhibit the activity of disaccharidases by preventing contact with the substrate (food). Irritating or toxic substances produced by yeast, bacteria, or parasites can damage the microvilli and destroy their enzymes.

Conditions associated with a deficiency of disaccharidases are celiac disease, malnutrition, cholera, gastroenteritis, diarrhea, irritable bowel syndrome, milk intolerance, soy intolerance, and Crohn's disease. Much documentation exists linking ulcerative colitis to lactase deficiency.

Cellulase

The body does not produce cellulase. Cellulase plays a valuable role by breaking down the soluble fiber (protective cellulose layer) found around all the cells in fruits and vegetables. Cellulase is liberated and begins its work when the cells are broken apart through chewing. While all raw fruits, vegetables and whole grains contain cellulase, high levels are found in vegetables, wheat and millet. Fruits such as apples, papaya, pears, and some melons also contain high levels of cellulase. Since the human body does not produce cellulase, chewing raw fruits and vegetables well releases the cellulase from the cells and aids in the digestion of these foods. Cooking vegetables and fruits will break down the cellulose layer but also destroys the enzymes (cellulase) contained in the food.

Cellulase has been shown to be able to the digest yeast-fungi responsible for yeast overgrowth syndrome.

The Overworked Pancreas

Studies show that when the diet consists of mostly cooked foods containing no enzymes, the pancreas will actually enlarge to keep up with the demand. This is called pancreatic hypertrophy. The significance of this is that the types of food eaten affect the health of the pancreas. When the pancreas must produce greater amounts of enzymes than normal, it enlarges. The same thing happens to your heart if it must pump blood through arteries that are clogged with cholesterol. Enlargement of an organ has long been associated with pathology. When laboratory mice are fed heat-treated or cooked food with no enzymes, their pancreases weigh two to three times as much as those of wild mice eating raw food.

The consequences of excess demand on the pancreas are described in the book *Victory over Diabetes*, by William H. Philpott, MD and Dwight K. Kalita, PhD - "An over stimulated pancreas follows the same general law that other over stimulated tissues and organ systems

A human weighing 140 pounds has a pancreas weighing approximately 85-95 grams. The pancreas of a sheep weighing 84 pounds is only 19 grams. If the sheep doubled its weight to 170 pounds its pancreas would still weigh only 38 grams, or less than half the weight of a human pancreas. The sheep eats all raw food – a high enzyme diet, needing less help from the pancreas.

The Law of Adaptive Secretion

The pancreas works according to the law of adaptive secretion. This means that enzymes are secreted by the pancreas on demand. The quantity and type of food determines the quantity and type of enzymes secreted. For example, a large, starchy meal of pasta will stimulate large amounts of amylase, whereas a steak will cause an abundance of protease to be secreted. In other words, there is specific secretion for specific foods. The pancreas will secrete only the types and amounts of enzymes it needs for the job at hand. It will not secrete more than necessary. However, when highly refined, cooked food is eaten, the food contributes no enzymes and the demand on the pancreas goes up. In 1943, Northwestern University established the law of adaptive secretion by experiments on rats. The amount of digestive enzymes secreted by the pancreas in response to carbohydrate, protein and fat was measured, and it was found that the quantity of each enzyme varied with the amount of the food it was to digest.

Besides enlargement, another condition called digestive leukocytosis results when cooked foods with no enzymes are ingested.

Digestive Leukocytosis

Digestive leukocytosis is an increase of white blood cells in the blood stream that occurs when certain types of foods are eaten. Leukocytosis, generally considered a pathological condition, can be observed in cases of infection, intoxication and poisoning. In 1930 Paul Kautchakoff, MD proved that leukocytosis can also be caused by ingesting cooked food. His findings were as follows: raw or frozen foods caused no increase in white blood cell count. common cooked foods caused a mild leukocytosis; pressure-cooked and canned foods caused a moderate leukocytosis; processed or highly refined foods (such as carbonated beverages, alcohol, vinegar, white sugar and white flour products) caused severe leukocytosis. Canned meat was the worst, bringing on a violent reaction equivalent to what might be seen in poisoning.

Why Does Digestive Leukocytosis Happen?

We know that white blood cells defend against invading organisms. The white blood cells are normally rich in enzymes. It is the enzyme activity that allows the white blood cell to engulf and destroy bacteria and viruses. The pancreas is a small organ, even in the enlarged state, and cannot itself produce all of the enzymes necessary to digest the food eaten, since that food averages up to five pounds a day. The pancreas can secrete and store a limited amount of enzymes. When the pancreas is over-stressed and over-stimulated, the white blood cells, or leukocytes, which normally have ample supplies of enzymes, are transported to the digestive tract to aid in the digestive process. This is a compensatory mechanism of the body in times of undue stress. Cooked food contains no enzymes, but the pancreas requires those missing food enzymes in conjunction with its stored digestive enzymes to digest food. When food enzymes are not present, the pancreas must call in the reserves - the white blood cells.

Enzymes are produced by all cells of the body. After a raw food meal there is no increase in the number of white blood cells in the blood stream. When cooked food is eaten, the whole body has to work much harder to produce and transport enzymes for the job of digestion. This leaves fewer enzymes to do metabolic work for the rest of the body. In nature, the pancreas was never intended to secrete 100% of the enzymes needed each time food is eaten.

How is Digestion Linked to the Immune System?

Here is the vital link. If white blood cells are giving up their enzymes to aid in the digestive process, they will have fewer enzymes for destroying bacteria and foreign invaders. With fewer enzymes, the leukocytes become sluggish and immobile. This is a mechanism by which you can impair your immune system every time you eat enzyme deficient food. The body's immune response is being mobilized to compensate for a lack of enzymes in the food. This can exhaust the immune system needlessly. There is a connection between the strength of the immune system and the body's enzyme levels. The greater the level of enzymes, the stronger the immune system and the healthier the person.

Enzymes can and do become depleted. Meyer and his associates at Michael Resse Hospital, Chicago, performed an experiment on the amylase of saliva. Two groups of subjects were used. In one group, the average age was 25 years and in another group the average age was 81 years. The amylase content in the saliva was 30 times greater in the younger group. These investigators found that young people can easily digest 50 grams of white bread in the mouth and stomach, while only 1% of it will be digested in the mouth and stomach of the older people. In general, high enzyme values are found in the tissues of young people and low values are found in older individuals with exhausted tissues. It is interesting to note that the enzyme content of body fluids is also low in chronic degenerative diseases, indicating tissue enzyme depletion.

Some of the symptoms of pancreatic enzyme deficiency are: gas after meals, bloating of the abdomen, skin problems, recurring headaches, muscle wasting and depression.

According to Dr. Philpott, when the pancreas is over-stimulated, the bicarbonate production is the first function to be inhibited. This is a function not given its proper place of importance, for it plays a major role in the acid-base balance of the body. Without sufficient bicarbonate production, the acid from the stomach cannot be adequately neutralized in the small intestine and the whole body can become acidic. The second function to suffer in pancreatic insufficiency is enzyme production. The consequence here, of course, is compromised digestion, particularly of protein. When protein cannot be broken down into amino acids, new enzymes cannot be built, as amino acids are the raw material required for enzyme production. Enzymes are protein compounds made from various combinations of amino acids. The body requires amino acids since approximately three-fourths of the solid parts of the body are protein, all built from amino acids.

The last function to be compromised in an over-taxed pancreas is insulin production. Insulin is best known as the substance needed by diabetics, but there is another aspect to diabetes. Diabetics also have been shown to have lowered blood levels of the enzyme amylase. The essential thing to remember is that the pancreas cannot be over-taxed without stressing the whole body.

Mary's Success Story

Mary, age 33, arrived at my office with a history of mental confusion, depression, suicidal tendencies, hyperactivity and inability to cope as a housewife and mother to three small children. She had been in and out of mental hospitals many times over the years. Examination revealed many digestive symptoms, and intolerance of yeast and nuts. She was also deficient in vitamin A. Additional foods and environmental allergies were suspected. Treatment consisted of enzyme therapy, a program for candidiasis, multiple minerals, a nutritional thyroid formula, a B-complex formula and vitamins A, C and E. Body organs were strengthened with specific reflex adjustments along the spine.

Because of her mental condition, this patient was unable to follow a treatment program consistently. Results were proportional to her compliance to the program. For example, Mary tested allergic to smoke but did not stop smoking. However, she did manage to follow the instructions enough to notice improvement. Although she was up and down a lot mentally, she recognized that she was getting better. Enzyme therapy seemed to particularly benefit her, as it appeared to halt the many reactions to foods and other substances

Since her treatment, Mary no longer has the suicidal tendencies or severe depression. Her general health has improved along with her digestion. She no longer requires hospitalization. All symptoms have cleared except for mild episodes of hyperactivity and some mental fog. This patient appears to be a fairly good example of the effects on the brain of food and environmental chemicals. Outlook for this patient is good if she continues to work to eliminate additional stressors to the body such as tobacco smoke, and if she continues her nutritional and enzyme therapy.

Evidence Links Low Enzyme Levels to Allergy

The concept of multiple enzyme deficiency rather than a single enzyme deficiency has not been studied in any depth. In cases of allergy, multiple enzyme deficiencies appear to prevail.

One way we know that low serum levels of enzymes induce allergy is through the research of Dr. Oelgoetz, an MD who performed experiments in the 1930s. When doses of pancreatic enzymes were given to patients with allergic symptoms and low serum enzyme levels, the serum enzyme levels returned to normal and the allergy subsided. Dr. Oelgoetz believed that when large, undigested food molecules enter the blood stream, the enzymes in the blood complete the process of digestion of the partially digested material. A low level of serum enzymes cannot do this.

Studies done by the Potter Metabolic Clinic in Santa Barbara, California showed good results in allergic disorders with the administration of enzymes. These results found bronchial asthma 88% improved, asthma induced by food 92% improved and eczema from food 83% improved.

Ray's Success Story

Violet, a woman in her sixties, was under treatment for carpal tunnel syndrome, which causes numbness of the fingers. She was excited about the help she had received and was free of her symptoms. She confided that she had only one problem left in her life, and that was her husband's snoring, which disturbed her greatly. I suggested that she bring her husband in for a check-up, which she did the following week.

Ray, also in his sixties, was in surprisingly good health, and only one abnormality was found during the examination. He was allergic to wheat. Ray was given nutritional plant enzymes to be taken prior to each meal and instructions to eliminate all wheat products from his diet for the next two weeks. Since his wife Violet did all the cooking for the family, she ensured that Ray ate no wheat. Within three days the snoring stopped.

Since one of the symptoms of allergy is a swelling of membranes, it appears that Ray must have experienced this swelling in the membranes along the roof of the mouth. As he breathed in while sleeping, the air rippled across these swollen membranes producing the loud snoring noise.

After about a month, while continuing to take his enzymes, Ray was able to include wheat in his diet again without a return of the snoring.

Facts about Cooked Foods

Many doctors still dispute the fact that diet is related to any kind of disease. But how could diet not be involved? In order for a human cell to survive, it needs the correct pH, temperature and supply of oxygen, minerals and nutrients. Nutrients can come only from diet. If these needs of the cell are not met, changes to the cell occur. If enough cells change, tissues begin to change, then organs. Organ changes bring on functional changes with far reaching effects in the body. Volumes have been written on how nutrients are related to the common illnesses of the day, especially chronic degenerative diseases such as heart disease, arthritis, diabetes, cancer and allergies. In 1982, the National Academy of Sciences estimated that 60% of women's cancers and 40% of men's cancers are related to diet. The most common cancers in this case are breast and uterine cancer, prostate and gastrointestinal cancer. With all the research available, it is becoming more and more apparent that diet indeed is a major factor in disease.

Doctors from around the world who have studied this situation have all come to the same startling conclusion – that cooked or heat-treated foods contribute to physical degeneration and disease. Ill health may not be acute, as seen in infectious disease, but may take a more insidious form such as fatigue, generalized aches and pains, ulcers, gastritis, arthritis, allergies and a shortened life span.

Cooking foods can convert the proteins into new forms which are either toxic or less digestible than the raw form. This stresses the digestive organs to produce more and more enzymes. In our diets, we have few sources of raw protein that contain the enzyme protease. We toast our nuts; we cook our meat and eggs, and we pasteurize our milk and dairy products. Yet, it has been shown that raw protein is more easily digested than the coagulated, cooked form.

In natural food, fat accompanies protein. Lipase is the enzyme that is normally found in fat. Once fat is cooked, the lipase is destroyed so that your body must now produce the lipase needed. Lipase is normally produced in lesser quantity than other digestive enzymes. Eating lipase-deficient fats is a potential source of stress for the digestive tract.

When lipase is deficient, fat contained in foods may be absorbed through the intestinal wall in a less digested, adulterated form. While circulating, this fat can diminish or choke off the amount of oxygen reaching the tissues and cells.

Since fat accompanies protein in foods, few raw fats are consumed. Therefore, minimal lipase enzyme is supplied from the diet. The fact that the human body has been able to adapt to some degree to denatured, cooked food is a miracle in itself. It is no accident that restorative or health-building diets have historically all been raw food diets including raw fruit and vegetable juices. These are the builders of the body because of their enzyme and nutrient content. They allow the digestive tract to rest and they contribute enzymes, which results in strengthening of the immune system.

Research done in Europe on cooked foods was reported in the book *Fats and Oils* by Udo Erasmus: "When cooked food is eaten, a defense reaction occurs in the tissues of the stomach and digestive tract. This reaction is similar to the reaction we find in infections and around tumors and involves the accumulation of white blood cells, swelling and a fever-like increase of temperature of the stomach and intestinal tissues."

Dr. M. Ted Morter, Jr. describes, from a chemical standpoint, what cooking does to food. He explains that the chemical bonds that hold compounds (such as foods) together are not all the same. Organically bonded molecules are loosely held together and easily broken. Inorganic or ionic bonds are tightly held together and not easily broken. Enzymes during digestion must break these bonds in order to make use of the elements in food. Dr. Morter reports, "When you heat covalent-bonded foods to more than a 130° F, bonds that are naturally weak are made stronger. As with strong ionic bonds, heat-strengthened bonds can't be broken easily, if at all. The elements are no longer as readily accessible for assimilation."

Animals in the wild eat only raw foods with loosely bonded molecules that are easy to digest and assimilate. Wild animals do not have the high incidence of chronic degenerative disease as do humans, unless they are domesticated and fed a heat-treated diet, or unless they are exposed to environmental chemicals and pollutants.

Dr. Marshal Mandell, in his book *Five Day Allergy Relief System,* states that "Substances are formed from foods during the cooking process that are totally alien to the human system and what it was designed to handle. Heating sugar creates foreign substances and caramelizes it, making tars. Browning meat creates tars all over the meat. Nothing like these tars exists in nature. And once proteins and carbohydrates and fats are heated they turn into substances that are alien to the human body."

In his book *Victory Over Diabetes* Dr. Philpott states, "Cooking food above 118° F destroys digestive enzymes. When this happens, the pancreas, salivary glands, stomach and intestines must all come to the rescue and furnish digestive enzymes to break down all those substances. To do this repeatedly the body must rob, so to speak, enzymes from other glands, muscles, nerves and the blood to help in its demanding process. Eventually the glands, and this includes the pancreas, develop deficiencies of enzymes, because they have been forced to work harder due to the low level of enzymes found in cooked food."

Dr. Philpott supports this idea with a study done at the University of Minnesota. Rats were given an 80% cooked food diet for 155 days. When examined, the pancreatic weight of the rats had increased by 20% to 30 %. There was a simultaneous decrease of digestive enzyme secretion.

In study after study done on animals where one group is fed cooked food and the other group is fed raw food, the results are the same. The group receiving cooked food demonstrates illness and deteriorates faster. Attempts to live on the wrong kinds of fuel burden the organs and tissues beyond their capacity to maintain health.

The Most Famous Studies on Cooked Food

Dr. Francis M. Pottenger, Jr., performed the most famous studies ever done comparing cooked food versus raw food between 1932 and 1942 - on cats. Pottenger's studies spanned ten years of cat generations and involved 900 cats. There is no similar experiment in current medical literature. Dr. Pottenger concludes that, "Normal cats on a raw food cod-liver oil diet, show no evidence of allergy or hypothyroidism and their offspring, generation after generation, show no evidence of allergy or hypothyroidism. The incidence of these deficiency problems corresponds with the introduction of cooked foods. In giving cats cooked meat and milk they develop all kinds of allergies. They sneeze, wheeze and scratch. They are irritable, nervous and do not purr. First deficient generation allergic cats produce second generation kittens with greater incidence of allergies. And by the third generation the incidence is almost 100%. When second generation allergic animals are bred after being returned to an optimum raw food diet, their allergic symptoms begin to diminish and by the fourth generation, some cats show no evidence of allergy."

The second and third generation of cats eating cooked meat showed abnormal respiratory tissues with edema, bronchitis and pneumonitis prevalent. Skin lesions and allergies were frequent and progressively worse from one generation to another.

The intestinal tracts of several hundred normal and deficient adult cats were compared at autopsy. Measurements were taken of the lengths of the gastrointestinal tracts. In a normal cat fed a raw diet, the intestinal tract was approximately 48 inches long. In the allergic cats the intestinal tracts could measure as long as 72 to 80 inches. These elongated tracts lacked tissue tone and elasticity. Based on his clinical experience and years of experiments Dr. Pottenger states, "We do know that ordinary cooking denatures proteins rendering them less easily digested. Probably certain albuminoids and globulins are physiologically destroyed. All tissue enzymes are heat labile and so destroyed. Vitamin C and some members of the B-complex are injured by the process of cooking and minerals are made less soluble by altering their physiological states."

Three indications that cooked foods are inferior are:

1. Pancreatic hypertrophy
2. Digestive leukocytosis
3. Loss of enzymes and nutrients.

In judging what is an adequate diet, just looking at calories, protein, carbohydrates, fats, vitamins, minerals and fiber are not enough. Availability of nutrients and enzyme content must also be considered, and the diet should be shown to sustain health generation after generation. Presence or absence of degenerative disease and length of life must also be considerations.

Food enzymes contained in raw foods can be absorbed by the human digestive tract, stored in the body and used at a later time. The fact that enzymes can be absorbed through the intestinal tract has been proven through numerous experiments. For instance, the oral use of proteolytic enzymes for sports injuries has been documented extensively. In the book *Enzyme Therapy*, Max Wolf, MD and Carl Ransberger, PhD relate an experiment using enzymes tagged with radioactive dye and given to rabbits. The active enzyme molecules were later recovered in the serum, liver, kidney and urine. Enzymes are absorbed from the intestine into the lymph system and later stored in the liver and spleen. There is evidence that enzymes are circulated and secreted over and over. Therefore, they have the potential to be used more than once before being "worn out" and excreted in the urine. By eating raw foods you help replenish the body's stores of enzymes by lowering the demand for enzymes from the digestive organs. Dr. Howell considers enzymes to be the "true yardstick of vitality." The more enzymes, the longer the life – the fewer the enzymes, the sooner disease, old age and death result.

What is the Body's Primary Response to Inflammation?

The body's primary response to inflammation is through the immune system, which uses increased amounts of enzymes during the inflammatory stage. Deficiencies of enzymes can prolong inflammation and delay healing. It has been shown that healing times can be reduced by up to 50% by the oral administration of proteolytic enzymes. The immune system also uses enzymes to break down microthrombi and fibrin clots, which aids in blood flow and waste removal to an injured area.

Donna's Success Story

Donna, age 37, appeared to be allergic to many things when I first saw her in my office. She stated that when she ate something to which she was allergic she would have an anaphylactic shock reaction. These reactions were preceded by dizziness, vomiting and severe abdominal pain. As a precaution, she carried epinephrine and a syringe in her purse for emergencies. Some of the foods she had previously reacted to included lettuce, cabbage, onions, peas, beans, walnuts, mustard, MSG (monosodium glutamate), shellfish, all grains, chocolate and tomatoes.

Examination of this patient revealed numerous allergies, hiatus hernia and structural misalignments. In addition she was suffering from a severe Candida overgrowth infection. Donna was given an herbal liquid formula to help heal the intestinal lining; a B-complex formula with chromium; Lactobacillus acidophilus to help reculture the bowel; an adrenal formula; an anti-Candida formula, and pancreatic enzymes. She received chiropractic adjustments once a week.

Donna was an intelligent woman eager to follow instructions. She responded well from the beginning. She had excellent follow-through on the diet and supplement program, and was prudent and knowledgeable about food choices. Her body strengthened rapidly and within two months she was able to expand her diet. After four months she had no further food reactions and was feeling great all the time. Her energy level was vastly improved.

After six months of treatment she was able to eat everything without reactions, except she was afraid to try a salad. Six months later she fi-

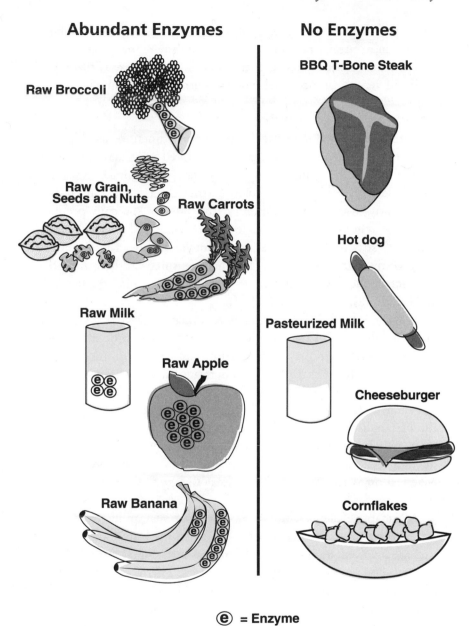

Abundant Enzymes

Raw Broccoli

Raw Grain, Seeds and Nuts

Raw Carrots

Raw Milk

Raw Apple

Raw Banana

No Enzymes

BBQ T-Bone Steak

Hot dog

Pasteurized Milk

Cheeseburger

Cornflakes

ⓔ = Enzyme

Raw foods are enzyme-rich

Figure 2. **Enzyme Content of Foods**

nally got up her nerve to eat a salad and was delighted when "nothing happened." At this time she did not require any nutrient supplements other than concentrated plant enzymes. In the three years that I followed the case, she never had another recurrence of anaphylactic shock.

Enzymes and Longevity

Eating more food than necessary for body functions uses up vast quantities of enzymes. This was demonstrated with an experiment done on rats. One group having unrestricted food intake lived 483 days. The other group with partially restricted food intake lived 894 days, nearly twice as long. Consider this: 50% of the daily production of protein in the body is made into enzymes and a major part of this is digestive enzymes. Lowering the intake of cooked foods means less digestive enzymes are used. This helps ensure that there are sufficient metabolic enzymes at work to keep the body running efficiently and healthfully.

Only one kind of food contains enzymes – raw food. A diet of 70% raw food and 30% everything else is a vast improvement over the enzyme-deficient diet that the majority of people consume. Statistics show that fewer than 10% of Americans eat two servings of fruit or three servings of vegetables per day. 50% eat no vegetables at all.

Vitamin B6 is a precursor to at least 50 enzymes and is needed for the metabolism of all amino acids. Enzymes are built from amino acids, which makes vitamin B6 a very essential part of enzyme production. Trace minerals must also be present for enzyme production. Magnesium is the mineral in greatest demand. Clinical Ecology states,

Maladaptive allergic and allergic-like reactions can likely be characterized by enzymatic deficiencies and when the immunological tissues are involved, antibodies are formed as a last stand at organismic survival. Nutrients are precursors to enzymes. Therefore, cellular malnutrition is the basis of these maladaptive reactions.

There are three ways to increase the enzyme content of your body.

1. Eat less food in general.
2. Eat more raw food.
3. Supplement with nutritional plant enzyme capsules.

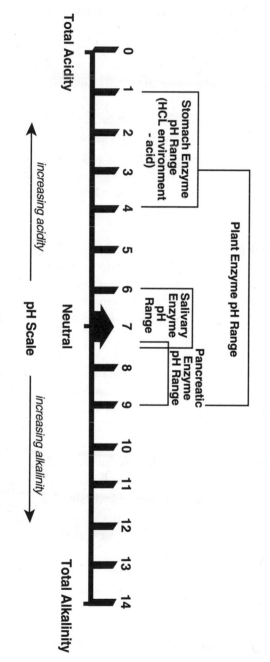

Figure 3. **Active Plant Enzyme pH Range**

Supplemental Plant Enzymes

When enzymes are lacking, illness results. Conversely, enzyme research has demonstrated that by taking supplemental enzymes orally on a daily basis, a person can help ensure digestion of food, elimination of toxic metabolites and environmental contaminants, reduce injury and pain following athletic activity and enhance healing following injury. Other benefits include reducing the likelihood or onset of degenerative conditions and allergies as well as slowing down aging.

Nutritional plant enzymes are safe and do not impair or impede the body's own production and metabolism of its own enzymes. Gastric ulcer is the only known condition in which nutritional plant enzymes should not be used.

Facts about Enzymes

- Enzymes are required for vitamins and minerals to work in the body. Vitamins and minerals are coenzymes and cannot perform work without the required enzyme. While vitamins and minerals are often given the credit, it is the enzymes that are performing behind the scenes.
- Enzymes found naturally occurring in food help in the digestive process. The importance of this role has not been appreciated. When foods containing enzymes are consumed, fewer enzymes are required to be produced by the body.
- Enzymatic activity is necessary and responsible for every biochemical reaction that occurs in living tissues.
- Food enzymes digest food before stomach acid is secreted and before the digestive tract must begin the process of digestion. Supplemental enzymes taken prior to a meal will simulate this action, thus ensuring more complete digestion without burdening the digestive system.
- Enzymes help to deliver nutrients to the body, even when the digestive tract is compromised and cannot function well.
- Enzymes found in foods are essential nutrients. Supplemental enzymes put back into the food the enzymes that are lost due to cooking and other food processing.
- When enzyme deficient, processed or cooked food is eaten, it can sit in the stomach for up to an hour with very little digesting taking

place. It takes the stomach up to an hour to secrete sufficient hydrochloric acid to initiate enzymatic action.

• Studies clearly show that enzymes are biochemically active and therefore can be exhausted and become deficient in the human body.

• Supplemental enzymes taken with a meal will digest food. Enzymes taken between meals on an empty stomach will be absorbed into the bloodstream and incorporated into the work of the body (metabolic enzymes).

• Nutritional enzyme supplements replenish enzyme losses due to diet, lifestyle, aging, illness and overeating.

Are Supplemental Enzymes Destroyed by the HCL in the Stomach?

This is a common misconception. HCL is not constantly present in the stomach. Following a meal, it takes 30 to 60 minutes for the stomach to concentrate sufficient HCL to initiate enzyme activity. HCL production occurs in response to stretching of the stomach wall by the presence of food. When supplemental enzymes are taken prior to a meal, they have up to an hour to work before the pH of the stomach becomes acid enough to deactivate them. When supplemental enzymes are taken between meals, the stomach is empty and there is no acid production.

How Fast Do Enzymes Work?

Enzymes are capable of working very fast when conditions of temperature, pH, and substrate are right. The slowest known enzyme, lysozyme, which helps destroy bacteria, can process about 30 substrate molecules per minute, or 1 substrate molecule every 2 seconds. By contrast, the enzyme carboanhydrase processes around 36 million substrate molecules in one minute.

How Long do Enzymes Last?

When an enzyme shows signs of wear and tear, it is broken down and replaced by a newly produced enzyme of the same type. Some enzymes have a life span of twenty minutes, while others may remain active for several weeks before they are replaced.

Supplemental enzymes are taken prior to a meal; they have up to an hour to work on the food before the peak of the HCL production.

Can My Body Become Dependent on Supplemental Enzymes?

When plant enzymes are supplemented prior to a meal, they have up to an hour to digest the food in the stomach before the stomach's enzymes go to work. Supplemental enzymes have the effect of resting the overworked and stressed digestive organs, which often are under-producing enzymes when symptoms are present. After a recuperative period, the digestive organs are able to produce more enzymes than before.

What Causes Gas and Bloating?

Gas and bloating can be caused by inadequate HCL acid in the stomach; decreased bile flow to emulsify the food; enzyme deficiency or lessened enzyme production; insufficient bicarbonate secretion by the pancreas; inadequate sugar-digesting enzyme production by the small intestine; abnormal intestinal flora; normal intestinal flora acting on incompletely digested foods; and chronic overeating. Regardless of the cause, the bottom line is that digestion is compromised in some way.

How Can Supplemental Enzymes be Used to Boost Immune System Function?

Proteases have been shown to be absorbed through the intestine in substantial quantities where they enter the bloodstream and bind to serum proteins. Tissues involved with immune function can then utilize them.

Supplementing enzymes between meals allows for this absorption to take place and contributes to immune system function.

Nutritional plant enzymes have been shown to have advantages over other forms of enzyme supplementation.

10 Reasons to Choose Nutritional Plant Enzymes

1. Although enzymes have very specific pH ranges, nutritional plant enzymes have a broad pH range (from 3 to 9) and are

the only enzymes that are capable of working throughout the entire digestive tract. They work in both acid and alkaline environments, ensuring more complete digestion of foods even when the digestive tract is incompetent. In contrast, animal enzymes such as pancreatin have a narrow pH range (from 7 to 9), and work only in an alkaline environment.

2. Enzymes have very specific temperature requirements. Nutritional plant enzymes have their greatest activity range between 95° and 105° F which means that their greatest activity is in the range of normal body temperature. In contrast, the enzyme bromelain works best in a temperature range of 120° to 160° F, which is well above body temperature. Papain has a similar action in temperature range. This limits the ability of these enzymes to do work since the human body temperature is not near their peak capacity.

3. Plant enzyme capsules are a better choice than tablets. Enzymes lose from 40% to 60% of their potency by being compressed into tablet form.

4. During inflammation, the immune system uses increased quantities of enzymes and therefore has an increased need for enzymes. Studies show that oral supplementation of proteolytic enzymes can reduce healing times by up to 50%.

5. Nutritional plant enzymes work to digest food in the stomach in the 45 to 60 minutes it takes the stomach to concentrate sufficient hydrochloric acid to initiate enzyme activity. 30% to 60% of the food can be digested during this time, sparing the digestive organs. Because the pancreas works on demand, food that is more completely digested when it reaches the small intestine will require less enzymes from the pancreas, taking stress off of that organ.

6. Nutritional plant enzymes replace enzymes that are lost when food is cooked and processed. The digestive activity of plant enzymes closely resembles that of food enzymes and will effectively digest protein, carbohydrates, fat, and fiber. In contrast, pancreatin can only break down three of these food categories: protein, carbohydrate, and fat.

7. Nutritional plant enzymes work in the stomach prior to the stomach beginning its own digestive process. They reduce the amount of hydrochloric acid that must be supplied.

8. Supplemental pancreatic enzymes and pepsin have virtually no effect on correcting poor protein digestion in the stomach caused by a lack of hydrochloric acid because pepsin is not active when hydrochloric acid is absent. Pancreatin can only work in an alkaline environment and cannot function in the stomach. Nutritional plant enzymes digest protein regardless of whether the stomach produces too little or too much hydrochloric acid.

9. Nutritional plant enzymes do not function like antacids, which turn off all digestion and put the entire stress of digestion on the pancreas. Plant enzymes relieve and correct indigestion by breaking down the foods that the incompetent digestive tract is unable digest.

10. Nutritional plant enzymes work early enough in the digestive process to relieve stress on the pancreas, by requiring less enzyme production, since enzymes are only secreted as needed. Supplemental pancreatin must wait until it is in the alkaline fluids of the small intestine for its digestive action. As this occurs late in the digestive process, the pancreas must still produce all the enzymes needed to completely digest the food.

12

Acid-Base Balance is Essential

O ne of the most important but least understood conditions affecting the healing process is the acid-base balance of the body. Not only is the proper pH of the body essential to healing, it is essential to prevent further allergic reactions.

Guyton's Textbook of Medical Physiology states that regulation of the pH of the body is one of the most important aspects of homeostasis.

What is pH?

pH is a measure of the acidity or alkalinity of a substance on a scale which runs from 0 to 14 with 7 being neutral. Neutral is neither acid nor alkaline. Zero is totally acid and 14 totally alkaline. In between are varying degrees of acidity and alkalinity.

The blood in the human body is at a pH of 7.4, which is slightly alkaline. If the pH of the blood were to make as small a change as to 6.8, which is barely acid, severe consequences, such as coma, would result. The heart would relax and then stop beating. If the pH of the blood were to increase to just 8.0, tetanic convulsions would occur and the heart would cease to beat. According to *Guyton's Textbook of Medical Physiology*, "Only slight changes in hydrogen ion concentration from the normal value can cause marked alteration in the rate of chemical reactions in the cells, some being depressed and others accelerated."

Since life-threatening conditions can occur with only small changes in the blood pH, the body will do whatever is necessary to maintain a constant blood pH of 7.4. Survival depends on the blood remaining at the slightly alkaline pH of 7.4.

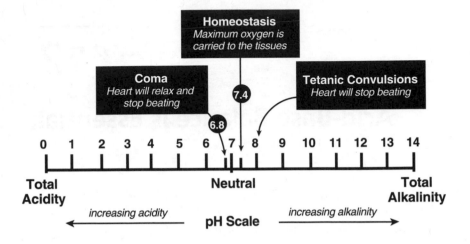

The blood must remain within a narrow pH range around 7.4.
The body gives blood pH priority over other body functions:
The heart will stop beating if the blood pH lowers to 6.8 or rises to 8.0.

Figure 4. **Blood pH Range**

When the blood shows a slight degree of acidity, a greater swing toward acidity at the cellular level usually occurs. As the blood is pushed by stimuli in an acid direction, it will buffer this acid with alkalizing minerals from other tissues. These minerals include potassium, sodium, calcium and magnesium. Once used, these minerals can be replaced in the body only by foods, particularly the alkaline fruits and vegetables.

Fruits and vegetables contribute minerals to your body in the following manner. Organic acids, such as those found in citrus fruits and most vegetables, contain the alkalizing minerals: sodium, potassium, calcium and magnesium. When oxidized, these organic acids become carbon dioxide and water, which are eliminated through the lungs and kidneys. The alkaline minerals remain behind and neutralize body acids (acid waste from cell metabolism). This is why most fruits and vegetables are considered to be alkaline-forming foods. They are mineral donors.

The sodium that the body requires cannot come from the sodium found in table salt (sodium chloride). The reason is that table salt has tight ionic bonds which are difficult for the body to break apart.

Table salt has been heated to over 500 degrees F in the refining process, making those bonds even tighter. The body can easily use sodium with loose covalent bonds, such as is found in raw fruits and vegetables. These foods are the main suppliers of sodium to the body.

The typical recommendation to cut back on salt is good advice when it comes to processed foods and table salt. However, sodium from natural fruits and vegetables is an essential nutrient and plays a major role in the body. Sodium drives the sodium-potassium pump in every cell of the body. The main function of this pump is to produce energy in the form of ATP (adenosine triphosphate). Without sufficient sodium, energy production decreases. Fatigue is the result. Sodium and potassium are necessary for this vital body function, as well as for neutralizing the acids of the body.

In allergic conditions, slight changes in acid-base metabolism occur. Excess acidity depletes the body's stores of minerals. Having fewer minerals lowers the body's ability to make enzymes since minerals are necessary for enzyme production and for carrying electrical currents in the body. Eating more alkalizing foods such as fruits and vegetables helps restore minerals to the body and promotes healing.

In addition, excess acidity causes the activity of the cells to slow down. When this happens, fatigue results. Fatigue is the number one symptom in most degenerative conditions including allergy. When the cells are impaired, the ability of each cell to produce energy is diminished. How do our modern diets relate to acid-base balance? We find some rather shocking news. In the last 50 years fruit and vegetable consumption has decreased by 40% to 45%. At the same time fat, salt and sugar consumption has increased by 100%. Whole grain consumption has decreased substantially, while consumption of bakery goods has increased by 70%. These changes are due to the increased production and availability of refined, processed and fast foods.

Fruits and vegetables are the body's main source of minerals or alkaline elements. A diet lacking fruits and vegetables and containing excess meat, fat and refined products will constantly push the body pH toward the acid state. This type of diet does three things:

1. It supplies many acid-forming factors.
2. It fails to contribute alkaline-forming elements.

3. It uses up the body's stored minerals by requiring excessive quantities of them to neutralize acids.

Stimulating the body continuously in one direction has the effect of eventually exhausting the body systems. The body will then change its functions in order to adapt to the new situation. These adaptations in function eventually lead to degenerative changes in tissues, organs and bony structures.

Diet is the largest single stimulus to the body's biochemical balance or homeostasis. Whatever you put in the body, the body must deal with, and you can drive your body in either an acid or alkaline direction over a period of time. Dr. M. Ted Morter Jr. explains, "Disease is a by-product of lowered resistance. Lowered resistance is a by-product of an unfavorable internal environment. An unfavorable internal environment is brought about principally by putting the wrong things into the body for it to work with." Let's look at each of these wrong things: excess protein, excess fat and refined foods.

Excess Protein

The average American eats 80 to 125 grams of protein per day. This is twice the Recommended Daily Allowance (RDA) for protein intake. The RDA recommends 63 grams for mature males and 50 grams for mature females. The RDA recommendations for protein have decreased over the last 20 years and many doctors feel the RDA for protein could be even lower.

Guyton's Textbook of Medical Physiology tells us that 20 to 30 grams of protein replaces the protein used up by the body daily. It suggests that an average person can maintain normal protein stores with a daily intake of 30 to 55 grams. Protein is continuously being broken down and re-synthesized by the body. The Recommended Dietary Allowances (RDA), 10th edition, states, "Several times more protein is turned over daily within the body than is ordinarily consumed indicating that re-utilization of amino acids is a major factor of the economy of protein metabolism." The same volume tells us that protein deficiency, besides being rare, does not occur in an isolated condition, but rather as a consequence of total calorie deprivation. In other words, it is difficult to have a protein deficiency in the absence of total starvation.

Some people feel they need to increase protein intake to compensate for vigorous exercise. This is not true according to the RDA... "There is little evidence that muscular activity increases the need for protein except for the small amount required for the development of muscles during physical conditioning." The RDA further states that, "In the view of the margin of safety in the RDA no increment is added for work or training." The authors of the RDA have already added an extra amount of protein to what studies show is actually required, making it unnecessary to include more protein for work. This "margin of safety" means that extra protein for work has already been included even though you may be sedentary.

How much is 30 Grams of Protein?

Food Source	Protein Content
Almonds (4 ounces)	20 grams protein
Beef burrito	25 grams protein
Big Mac(tm)	25 grams protein
Cheddar cheese (4 ounces)	28 grams protein
Cheese, American (4 ounces)	24 grams protein
Chicken nuggets (6)	20 grams protein
Chicken, broiled (4 ounces)	33 grams protein
Egg (1)	6 grams protein
Flounder, broiled fresh (4 ounces)	27 grams protein
Hamburger (4 ounces)	20 grams protein
Kidney beans, boiled (1/2 cup)	6 grams protein
Pepperoni pizza (two slices)	26 grams protein
Pinto beans, boiled (1/2 cup)	7 grams protein
Taco salad with the shell	34 grams protein
Tofu, firm (1/2 cup)	20 grams protein
Whole milk (1 cup)	8 grams protein

The acids produced from excess protein must be neutralized to prevent them from harming the body. In accomplishing this, the alkaline minerals: sodium, calcium and potassium are used. If excess protein must be continuously neutralized over a long period of time, the body's alkaline reserve is depleted. So what should be done? The message here is not to stop eating protein altogether. Protein is absolutely essential for health. It is the excess protein that creates problems and toxicity in the body, stressing alkaline reserves. You must know how much protein you are consuming and keep the amount to a healthful level.

As you can see, only a small amount of protein is actually required daily. How many people sit down to an eight-ounce (64 grams) or 12 ounce (96 grams) steak for dinner and consume that in only one meal? Perhaps they also had bacon (6 grams per 3 slices) and eggs (12 grams per 2 eggs) for breakfast and a hamburger (24 grams) for lunch. That would be a total of 138 grams.

Excess protein can create dangerous conditions in the body. Most animal proteins supply sulfur and phosphorus. Phosphorus is abundant in animal-source foods and can produce poisonous acid. When animal protein is metabolized, sulfur and phosphorus form sulfuric and phosphoric acid, which must be neutralized by the alkaline body minerals before the kidneys can excrete them. This is the reason animal foods are considered to be acid forming foods.

Furthermore, excess protein breaks down to produce urea, which has a diuretic effect causing both water and valuable minerals such as calcium, sodium and potassium to be lost in the urine. Since these minerals are alkaline-forming elements, the result of excess protein is to push the body toward the acid state.

Excess protein can also change the pH of the fluids surrounding the cells, thereby upsetting the osmotic balance of the cells. The osmotic balance is the pressure between the fluids on either side of the cell membrane. When the pH of these fluids changes water may flow into the cells. Protein synthesis inside the cell can be impaired by alterations of the pH of the fluid surrounding the cell.

All functions in the body are dependent upon the pH balance. However, of particular interest is how white blood cell production depends upon the acid-base balance. When the body is pushed towards the acid side, white blood cell production is lowered. This, of course, interferes with the immune system which relies on its white blood cells.

How does all this relate to allergy? *Clinical Ecology* tells us, "Maladaptive symptoms quickly develop when the pH is not optimum."

Monitoring pH at the time that maladaptive symptoms develop reveals that acidification is characteristic. Many allergic reactions not only occur in, but also help to create acid conditions in the body. *Clinical Ecology* goes on to say that it takes a very strong stimulus for a healthy person to develop symptoms.

A biologically healthy organism will develop symptoms on exposure to overwhelmingly strong stimuli. A biologically defective organism, due to an irritable or over-responsive central nervous system, will develop symptoms to normal or even subnormal stimuli.

Symptoms when the Body is in a Slightly Acid State.

Fatigue, pain, stomach pain, chest pain, frequent sighing, allergies, insomnia, water retention, arthritis, migraine headaches, low blood pressure, dry hard stools, alternating constipation and diarrhea, difficulty swallowing, burning in the mouth and/or under the tongue, bumps on the roof of the mouth or tongue and aches and pains on arising which improve as the day goes on

Symptoms when the Body is in a Slightly Alkaline State

Sore muscles, creaking joints, bursitis, bone spurs, drowsiness, hypertension, hypothermia (low body temperature), edema, allergies, night cramps, asthma, chronic indigestion, night coughs, vomiting, menstrual problems, hard dry stools, prostatitis and skin itching. In the absence of major pathology, the primary cause of alkalosis is the taking of antacids for digestive complaints.

One study showed that when grain, which produces an acid residue in the body, was chewed 100 to 200 times per mouthful, the grain became alkaline by mixing with the alkaline salivary enzyme ptyalin and thus did not create acidity. The blood can most easily stay at the slightly alkaline pH of 7.4 when alkaline foods predominate in the diet. A blood pH of 7.4 creates a healing environment and regeneration at the cellular level. If you give the body what it needs, it can do the necessary repair. In general, fruits and vegetables are alkalizing and meats and grains are acidifying.

Excess Fat

Fats have an acidifying effect because excess fat tends to block oxygen from reaching the cells. With less oxygen, the sodium-potassium pump of the cell slows down and waste products start to accumulate in the cell. These waste products are acidic. In addition, excess fat is often incompletely broken down by the digestive tract and metabolism. This incomplete burning of fat produces acetic acid.

Refined Foods

White sugar and white flour products, candy, soft drinks, many drugs and processed foods are all acid-forming This is because they lack minerals and must rob minerals from body tissues in order to be metabolized.

As little as two teaspoons of refined white sugar is enough to change mineral relationships in the body. All minerals work in relation to one another, so changing those relationships means some minerals will be unavailable when needed.

Researchers have found that eating sugar increases the excretion of calcium in the urine. This alone can upset the mineral balance in the body. When sugar is eaten day after day and year after year, it stresses the balance or homeostasis of the body.

Other studies have shown that two teaspoons of sugar is enough to significantly decrease the number of white blood cells, leading to immune system suppression.

Alkaline-Forming and Acid-Forming Foods

Foods are determined to be acid forming or alkaline-forming according to the residue or ash they leave in the body. In the following list of common foods, notice that alkaline ash comes primarily from fruits and vegetables and acid ash comes primarily from meats, grains and refined carbohydrates. There is often confusion about acidic fruits such as lemons, oranges and grapefruit. These fruits have an alkalizing effect on the body because their acids are burned by the body, giving off carbon dioxide and water and leaving an alkaline mineral ash.

Alkaline-Forming Foods

Almonds
Apple
Apricot
Artichoke
Avocado
Banana
Beans
  Dried beans (most)
  Lima
  Navy
  Snap
Beets and beet greens
Berries:
  Blackberry
  Blueberry
  Gooseberry
  Raspberry
  Strawberry
Broccoli
Brussels sprouts
Buckwheat
Cabbage
Carrots
Cauliflower
Celery
Chard, Swiss
Cherry
Chestnuts
Chives
Coconut
Cucumber
Currants
Dandelion greens
Dates
Eggplant

Acid-Forming Foods

Bread
Cake
Cereals (processed)
Cornflakes
Crackers
Cranberry
Dairy products
Eggs
Fish:
  Codfish
  Haddock
  Salmon
  Sardines
  Tuna
Flours:
  White flour
  Whole wheat
Grains:
  Barley
  Corn
  Oats
  Rye
  Wheat
Lentils
Macaroni
Mayonnaise
Meats:
  Bacon
  Beef
  Chicken
  Corned beef
  Duck
  Ham
  Lamb
  Liver

149

Alkaline-Forming Foods

Endive
Garlic
Grapefruit
Grapes
Figs
Kale
Kohlrabi
Lemon
Lettuce
Lime
Mango
Melons:
  Cantaloupe
  Watermelon
Millet
Molasses
Mushrooms
Nectarine
Okra
Olives
Onion
Orange
Parsley
Peach
Pear
Peas
Peppers
Pineapple
Potato
Pumpkin
Radish
Raisins
Rhubarb
Rutabaga
Spinach

Acid-Forming Foods

Pork
Sausage
Turkey
Veal
Muffins
Nuts
Oatmeal
Pastries
Peanut butter
Peanuts
Persimmon
Pies
Plums
Prunes
Rice:
  Brown rice
  White rice
Shellfish:
  Clams
  Crab
  Lobster
  Oysters
  Scallops
  Shrimp
Soybeans
Spaghetti
Wheat germ

Neutral Foods with Acidifying Effect

Fats
Olive oil
Sugar syrups
Sugar, refined (white and brown)

Sprouts
Squash
Tangerine
Tomato
Turnip and turnip greens
Watercress
Yam

Your Cells in Allergy

Cells require specific conditions in order to stay healthy. If a cell's environment changes sufficiently and exceeds its capacity to maintain normal homeostasis, or balance, we get acute cell injury. If enough cells are injured, pathology results. It is said that we live or die at the cellular level. What conditions are necessary for cells to live in a healthy state?

An important condition is maintenance of the optimum pH of cells. Cellular enzymes, which control all functions of the cell, require a very narrow pH range. If the pH of the cell becomes too acid or alkaline, enzymatic function decreases and impairs survival of the cell. The pH also affects the function of insulin. Insulin moves glucose (a form of sugar) through the cell membrane to be burned for energy. If the extra-cellular fluids are not alkaline enough, glucose cannot enter the cell. The result is fatigue.

Cells must have a constant oxygen supply. When glucose enters the cell, it combines with oxygen in tiny organelles called mitochondria to produce ATP (adenosine triphosphate). ATP is the energy reserve or stored energy. When sufficient oxygen is available, between 32 and 36 moles of ATP per glucose unit are produced. If insufficient oxygen is supplied, as few as 3 moles of ATP per unit of glucose are produced. This is a considerable difference in ATP production, representing a much lowered energy production.

Research indicates that blood can carry the maximum amount of oxygen to your cells at the specific pH of 7.4. Therefore, any degree of acidosis or alkalosis would decrease the oxygen-carrying capacity of the blood and decrease energy production.

Diet is the greatest single stimulus affecting the blood, because eating is something that we do every day, several times a day. Two to five

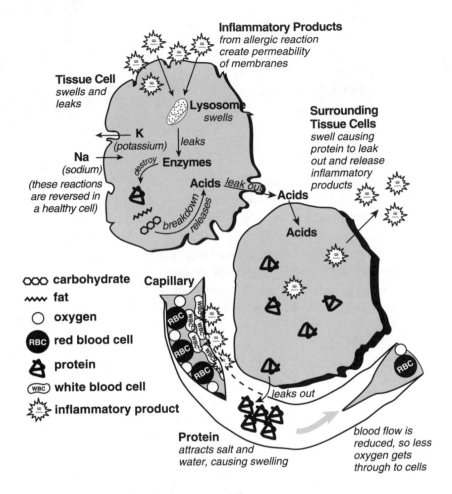

Figure 5. **The Cell Encounters Allergy**

pounds of food are metabolized daily. For the average person, two-thirds of the calories in the diet are from fat and sugar. When acid metabolites are produced faster than they can be neutralized, the blood pH changes and symptoms develop. Over-consumption of fats leads to acidosis by impeding the supply of nutrients and oxygen to the cells.

Minerals are also required for cells to function properly, and they must be balanced in proportion to one another. Sodium is found primarily in the fluids surrounding the cell while potassium is found primarily in the fluids inside the cell. If sodium decreases, fluid will flow into the cell, impeding cellular function. If sodium increases outside the cell, the fluid will flow from the cell to the surrounding tissue. Too much or not enough – both situations are undesirable. Balance is what is required.

What happens when an allergic reaction takes place in the tissues? How do cells react? Let's first look at the life of a normal cell.

The Life of a Normal Cell

We have in our bodies an estimated 70 to 100 trillion cells, each one like a little factory. Each cell is an expert in the processes of manufacturing, transportation and waste disposal. The cell depends on the blood stream and the extra-cellular fluids to bring it raw materials. It depends on the same fluids to carry away the waste. If the waste is not carried away quickly, its toxicity can damage the cell. If the proper raw materials are not supplied, cellular function can be compromised and damage can occur.

What kind of factory is the cell? It is an energy producer. For the cell to survive and thrive it must be able to generate enough energy to grow, to repair itself, to reproduce and to do the special work of the tissue it comprises. Oxygen, nutrients and intracellular enzymes are necessary for the cell to generate energy. Anything that compromises these three essentials threatens the survival of the cell. In addition, elimination of waste is essential. No cell can survive surrounded by its own refuse. The fluid surrounding the cell must remain clean, of proper mineral balance, of sufficient quantity and of constant pH.

Therefore, a proper nutrient supply linked with proper waste disposal and proper environment is the only way that the health of the cell can be maintained. If all of the cells are healthy there can be no allergy or any other disease in the body!

Likewise, the body as a whole has the same requirements as each cell. It must have oxygen and nutrients in order for it to grow, repair itself, reproduce and fulfill its function in the world. It must have an efficiently working waste disposal system (bowels, kidneys, lungs, and skin). This is the only way that health can be maintained.

What Happens to the Cell When it Encounters Allergy?

As cells become involved with an allergic reaction, a drama of events unfolds. When the allergic reaction takes place, cells release toxic products of allergic inflammation, which can penetrate the cell membranes of surrounding cells and cause the capillaries to become leaky. In the cells directly affected by allergic swelling, allergic inflammation manifests itself. It is the lysosome, the digestive organelle inside the cell, which swells. The membrane of the lysosome is disrupted, causing hydrolytic enzymes to pour out and destroy the protein, carbohydrate and fat within the cell. This creates acids which cause an acid pH inside the cell. We all know what acid rain does to our lakes. When an allergic reaction takes place, it is the equivalent of acid rain in the cells. The cell membrane leaks these acids into the fluids surrounding the cell. Potassium inside the cell is lost to the outside of the cell and sodium enters the cell, causing more swelling or edema.

As the body continues to respond to the allergic injury, protein leaks out of surrounding cells due to inflammatory toxins, which have caused capillary permeability (leakiness). The proteins coagulate outside the capillaries, causing the red blood cells to sludge, or slow down and stick together. The white blood cells stick to the capillary walls trying to plug the leaks. The result is that oxygen is inhibited from reaching the involved cells and acid waste products accumulate.

Lack of oxygen, slowed blood flow and increased acidity in the tissues together cause changes in the cell metabolism and lactic acid begins to build up, increasing acidity. The changes in cell metabolism can be mild to severe and they can be local or widespread. When enough tissue changes have occurred, symptoms develop. These can range all the way from slight fatigue to incapacitating illness, depending on the location and extensiveness of the injury.

13

Calcium Facts and Myths

Experts all agree that milk is the number one allergen. Medical textbooks on pediatrics also acknowledge the allergenicity of milk to babies and children. However, the first question that a patient will ask when told they are allergic to milk is, "Where will I get my calcium?" Although logical, this question is strange from the point of view that calcium is really no more or less important than many other minerals. For example, the mineral potassium is essential for every cell in the body. A severe deficiency will cause the heart to stop beating. Yet I seldom hear the question, "Where will I get my potassium?" This over-concern about calcium has been stimulated by radio, television and magazines, primarily in commercials and advertisements for milk, cheese and antacids. These sources teach that calcium is necessary for healthy bones and for prevention of osteoporosis. While this may be true, at the same time it has been oversimplified.

Osteoporosis is certainly a legitimate concern, especially for women. One in three women will lose enough bone minerals to cause fractures. This results in over 200,000 deaths annually. However, recent studies show that boosting calcium intake may not be the answer. There are many other factors involved.

Let's first explore some of the ways that calcium may be lost from the body. If you were in a boat that had sprung a leak, wouldn't it make sense to plug the hole first? Similarly, there are many ways that calcium is drained from the body.

Coffee, tea, soda pop and chocolate: Intake of caffeine causes increased calcium loss in the urine.

Refined sugar: Ingestion of sugar increases calcium loss through

155

urine. When foods containing calcium are taken with sugar, the absorption of usable calcium through the intestine is greatly reduced. Dr. J. B. Orr demonstrates that rickets, a calcium deficiency causing deformed bones in children, can be induced by the use of sweetened condensed milk. Many junk foods are a high source of sugar.

Phosphorus: Meat, grain and soft drinks have a high phosphorus content. Phosphorus binds with calcium. Therefore, when phosphorus is high in the blood, it can pull calcium from the bones. An excess intake of phosphorus results in secondary hyperparathyroidism (over-active parathyroid). A diet high in phosphorus has the same effect as a calcium deficiency. A cheeseburger with French fries and a glass of milk has 1,230 milligrams of phosphorus. The RDA of phosphorus for adults is 800 milligrams per day. On the other hand, too little phosphorus can also be detrimental. This is because calcium and phosphorus must be present in a specific ratio in order to work properly. Robert M. Giller, MD in his book *Medical Makeover* writes: "Sugar decreases the amount of phosphorus in the blood to such a degree that for two to five hours after a sugar snack, the body cannot sustain calcification."

Salt: Sodium, such as found in table salt increases urinary calcium excretion.

Fiber: A high fiber diet will decrease calcium absorption through the intestine. Many people add fiber to an already deficient diet, which can actually make their mineral absorption worse. This is due to the fact that minerals tend to bind to the fiber, becoming unavailable for use.

Vitamin D: Without vitamin D calcium cannot be utilized for bone formation. Vitamin D activates the absorption or transportation of calcium. Major food sources are eggs, liver and mushrooms. The sun is another source. Moderate sun exposure (approximately 20 minutes per day) is beneficial for most people.

Protein depletes calcium in two ways. High intake of protein causes loss of calcium through negative calcium balance. When we eat more protein than we need, the excess protein is broken down in the liver to urea. Urea has a diuretic action on the kidney which results in minerals, including calcium, being lost in the urine. Also, excess protein is acid forming, often pulling calcium from the bones to buffer the excess acidity. Most adults take in 100 to 125 grams of protein a day. John A. McDougall, MD reports on one long-term study which measured calcium balance and found that when 75 grams of protein a day was consumed along with 1400 milligrams of calcium, "More calcium was lost in the urine than was absorbed into the body from the diet (a negative calcium balance)." High protein consumption contributes more to depletion of calcium from bones than does a deficiency of calcium intake.

Other things that contribute to a loss of calcium from the body are smoking, alcohol consumption, a history of gastrointestinal surgery or malabsorption problems, and taking corticosteroid medications. It is apparent that body calcium is dependent upon habits, health and lifestyle. Simply taking the RDA of 800 mg of calcium daily will not necessarily ensure that you have enough calcium. You can increase or decrease the amount of calcium your body requires by the choices you make. Before concerning yourself with taking more calcium, it may be necessary to "plug the leaky boat."

Additionally, there are several myths about calcium, particularly surrounding the consumption of milk, which must be examined.

Calcium Myth One: Milk is Good for Everybody.

Fact: Milk is the number one allergic food. An estimated thirty-three million Americans are allergic to milk. Milk contains more than 25 different proteins that may induce allergic reaction. In addition, at least 60 million people in North America are lactose intolerant. Lactose intolerance is the inability to digest lactose, the sugar naturally present in milk. Lactase is the enzyme necessary to break down milk sugar. Most people stop manufacturing this enzyme between early childhood and adolescence. This is why 70% of the world population is lactase deficient. Perhaps this should be a tip-off that adults are not intended to drink milk. It is possible that this lack of lactase is not a deficiency, but a normal body condition. Lactose intolerance is the most common cause of gas, bloating, abdominal cramping and diarrhea.

This is an example of what can happen when only one enzyme is missing. New studies show that when one enzyme is deficient, there are usually other enzymes missing as well. We can only speculate about what happens in multiple enzyme deficiency. We do know, however, that if a food cannot be digested, its nutrients cannot be absorbed and utilized.

Milk may actually create a calcium deficiency. In a lactase deficient person, the lactose ferments in the intestine because it cannot be completely broken down. When it ferments it produces lactic acid, which is absorbed into the blood stream and subsequently binds with calcium and magnesium making these minerals potentially unavailable to the tissues. Remember, calcium is the most abundant alkaline mineral used by the body to counteract acidity. Calcium is used as a buffer to protect organs from the toxic effects of caffeine, alcohol and drugs.

Calcium Myth Two: Dairy Products Help Prevent Osteoporosis.

Fact: Milk loses 50% of its available calcium during pasteurization. Low fat and skim milk make calcium unavailable because fat is necessary for the proper transportation and absorption of calcium. According to a report in the *Journal of Nutrition* (February 1989), the calcium in cheese is even less available for utilization than the calcium in other dairy products. As far as osteoporosis is concerned, keep in mind that vegetarians have been shown to have higher bone density than meat eaters of the same age. Also, countries that consume the most dairy products have the most osteoporosis. Nutritionists agree that the best diet to prevent osteoporosis is a low protein, low fat, high complex carbohydrate diet that includes abundant fresh vegetables and fruit, whole grains and fresh raw seeds and nuts.

Calcium Myth Three: Calcium Supplementation Helps Prevent Osteoporosis.

Fact: This depends on whether you have plugged the leaky boat. Have you lowered your protein intake to the recommended level of 35 to 50 grams daily? Have you eliminated sugar, coffee, tea and soda pop from your diet? Are you eating abundant fresh fruits and vegetables? If so, calcium supplementation may not be necessary. However, if you wish to supplement, some forms of calcium are absorbed better than others. Huge doses are undesirable because less absorption takes place when too much calcium is taken at once.

Calcium Supplements and Absorption Rates

Calcium carbonate: 50% calcium ,used in many antacids

Calcium citrate: 50% calcium, probably the best absorbed calcium

Calcium gluconate: 9% calcium, usually well absorbed

Calcium hydroxapetite: 24% calcium, also very well absorbed.

Calcium lactate: 13% calcium People who are not allergic or intolerant to milk absorb calcium lactate, found in milk, best.

Calcium orotate and chelate: 10% calcium, usually well absorbed.

Bone meal and dolomite: lowest absorption and questionable because some brands have been shown to contain pollutants such as aluminum and lead.

If you are going to take a supplement, a formula of calcium combined with other minerals is the safest choice, so as not to deplete other minerals or upset the mineral balance. No mineral in the body works alone. Each affects the other. As we have seen, there are many factors to consider in relation to calcium.

Milk as a Source of Calcium

Milk is not necessarily the answer to obtaining enough calcium. If you are allergic to milk, it definitely is not the answer. If you cannot digest milk, you cannot absorb its calcium. The milk I described here is the homogenized, pasteurized product found in supermarket dairy cases. This is a processed food with its enzymes destroyed. It requires your body to donate an enormous amount of enzymes to digest it.

Fat free milk is not without problems either. When the fat is removed the same amount of milk is higher in protein, which may cause or contribute to a negative calcium balance. Fat free milk still contains allergenic proteins and indigestible sugars.

Unpasteurized raw milk contains an enzyme, which splits the calcium from the phosphorus it is bound to, making the calcium more available to the human body. Raw milk is also a high enzyme product, requiring far less of your own body's enzymes to digest it.

Sources of Calcium
It is possible to get enough calcium in your diet without using dairy products. The following list of non-dairy foods shows that daily calcium requirements can be met without using whole cow's milk, which contains only 288 mg of calcium per cup.

Seeds and Nuts (1 cup portions)
almonds	600 mg calcium
filberts (hazelnuts)	424 mg calcium
sesame seeds	2,200 mg calcium
sunflower seeds	260 mg calcium
walnuts	216 mg calcium

Nut Butters (3-ounce portions)
Almond butter	225 mg calcium
Cashew butter	36 mg calcium
Filbert (hazelnut) butter	159 mg calcium
Peanut butter	15 mg calcium
Sesame butter	843 mg calcium
Sunflower seed butter	99 mg calcium

Note: Peanut butter is not recommended as it delivers the least calcium and is the most allergenic.

Nut Milk
Nut Milk is a good substitute for cow's milk as it is very high in calcium and a good source of essential fatty acids, necessary for health. Nut milks can be used on cereals, in recipes, or for drinking from a glass. Nut milk made from two ounces of sesame seeds and two ounces of almonds will contain 712 mg of calcium per cup. Nut milk containing three ounces of sesame seed and two tablespoons of Barbados molasses will yield approximately 940 mg of calcium per cup. Since the calcium in nut milks has not been heated or cooked, it is highly absorbable and can be easily digested. Another way to add

calcium to foods is to sprinkle sesame seeds on cereals, salads, casseroles and all vegetable dishes.

Vegetables (1/2 cup portions)

Artichoke, 1 medium	47 mg calcium
Asparagus (six spears)	22 mg calcium
Avocado, 1 medium	19 mg calcium
Beans, Green	29 mg calcium
Broccoli	21 mg calcium
Cabbage	18 mg calcium
Carrot, 1 medium	19 mg calcium
Collard greens	74 mg calcium
Kale	47 mg calcium
Lamb's quarters	232 mg calcium
Mustard greens	52 mg calcium
Okra	50 mg calcium
Parsley	39 mg calcium
Peas	22 mg calcium
Spinach	16 mg calcium
Swiss chard	51 mg calcium
Turnip greens	53 mg calcium
Watercress	20 mg calcium

Molasses (1 tbsp.)

Blackstrap	137 mg calcium
Barbados	49 mg calcium

Beans and Rice (1 cup portions)

Brown rice	23 mg calcium
Garbanzo beans (chick peas)	80 mg calcium
Kidney beans	50 mg calcium
Navy beans	128 mg calcium
Pinto beans	82 mg calcium
Soybeans	460 mg calcium
Three bean salad	88 mg calcium
Tofu	258 mg calcium
Wild rice	30 mg calcium

Seaweed (3 1/2 oz portions)

Agar	54 mg calcium
Irish moss	72 mg calcium
Kelp	68 mg calcium
Wakame	150 mg calcium

14

Fats and Oils: Surprising Link to Allergy

F ats and oils are probably the most misunderstood and controversial of all the dietary nutrients. So much information and misinformation has become available about fats that it is difficult for interested people to sort out the facts. How fats relate to allergy has been even more of a mystery.

Why cholesterol, just one of many fatty substances has been disproportionately singled out as the culprit in diseases involving fats is beyond comprehension. With this focus on cholesterol, the majority of people are unaware of the effects of toxic trans-fatty acids and harmful free radicals, which have a proven record of damage to human tissues.

Since 75% of the North American population dies prematurely of diseases related to fats, learning which fats to use, which to avoid and what fats do in the body becomes an absolute prerequisite to maintaining good health. In addition, today's fats and oils have a surprising connection to allergy.

Fats are the only food group not absorbed into the blood from the intestinal lining. Instead, they are broken down into fatty acids and absorbed into the lymphatics. Here they are circulated and eventually enter the blood stream. Fats alone seldom trigger allergic reactions. Although milk is a highly allergenic food, butter seldom causes an allergic reaction. However, many commonly eaten fats pave the way for inflammatory or allergic reactions. This is why it is so important to identify these fats and eliminate them from the diets of people with allergies. There is no point in feeding inflammatory-type foods to an individual whose body is already inflamed with allergies.

There are only two fatty acids that are considered essential to life. They are essential because they cannot be manufactured in the body and must be obtained from the diet. These two fatty acids are called linoleic (LA or Omega 6) and linolenic (LNA or Omega 3). Sources of LA include safflower, sunflower, corn, soy and sesame oils. The best sources of LNA are flaxseed or hempseed oils. Both of these fatty acids play important roles in protecting your cardiovascular system and heart from atherosclerosis.

That is only one reason why these fatty acids are important. They are also converted into hormone-like substances in your body called prostaglandins. Prostaglandins act as messengers and regulate vital metabolic processes throughout the body. About 30 prostaglandins have been discovered to date. There are three major categories or families of prostaglandins. Prostaglandins act like a check and balance system in the body. For every action of one prostaglandin there is a prostaglandin that performs the opposite action. For example, if one prostaglandin were to turn on the water faucet, there would be another prostaglandin to turn it off. Keeping them in balance is important. Consider our water faucet prostaglandins; one prostaglandin turns on the water; but the other prostaglandin is disabled and cannot turn it off. The water overflows the sink. What if another prostaglandin comes along and turns on another faucet and the disabled prostaglandin still cannot turn it off? The whole house could be flooded. Similar events happen in your body when you eat the wrong kinds of fat.

To allergy sufferers the prostaglandins that play a role in controlling inflammation are the most important. For instance, LNA (Omega 3) helps control allergic manifestation in the skin in the form of eczema. Inflammation in the body is not always bad. It is a normal and natural part of the healing process. When you have a cut in the skin, it is the inflammatory process that calls the appropriate cells to the area to heal the wound. Inflammation out of control is destructive. Prostaglandins can either create inflammation or inhibit it. Inflammation running wild is part of allergic reactions. It can be controlled depending on what type of fat is fed to the body.

There are basically two kinds of fats, saturated and unsaturated. Saturated fat is solid at room temperature and comes mainly from animal sources. Unsaturated fat is liquid at room temperature and comes from vegetable sources. The fatty acid LA converts to the prostaglandin 1 family (called PG1) whose effects prevent inflammation, block allergic responses, and enhance the immune system. The fatty acid LNA converts to the prostaglandin 3 family (PG3), which also prevents inflammation and enhances the immune system. PG3 blocks the release of inflammatory products from the mast cells and basophils that are involved in allergic reactions.

The prostaglandin 2 family (PG2) has the opposite effect. It promotes inflammation, suppresses the immune system and stimulates the allergic response. PG2 is built from a fatty acid known as arachidonic acid. Sources of arachidonic acid are meat, milk and eggs. You can see at once that most people eat far more meat, milk and eggs than they do flaxseed oil. That is why in some allergic individuals it is necessary to limit or eliminate those foods in order to bring inflammation under control. In other words, removal of these foods from the diet stops feeding the inflammatory pathway. (See Figure 6.)

Addition of flaxseed or hempseed oil to the diet feeds the anti-allergic, anti-inflammatory pathway. Did you ever notice a big flare-up of symptoms one to three days after eating a big steak dinner or a pizza (meat and milk products)? Or perhaps you are eating meat, milk and eggs on a daily basis and have continual or chronic inflammation. These arachidonic acid foods load up your cells with inflammatory substances. When the allergic reaction takes place, the cell membrane breaks releasing these inflammatory substances and causing tissue damage. It makes sense for people who are prone to allergy to restrict foods that feed inflammatory reactions.

Leukotrienes are one substance made from arachidonic acid. They are 1,000 to 10,000 times more inflammatory than histamine. Leukotrienes are often involved in allergic reactions, especially asthma.

It sounds simple. Cut back or eliminate foods that encourage inflammation and add the inflammation-fighting oils into your diet. But there is more. Fats are converted to fatty acids and prostaglandins by a series of steps that involves enzymes, vitamins and minerals. If

Important Pathways

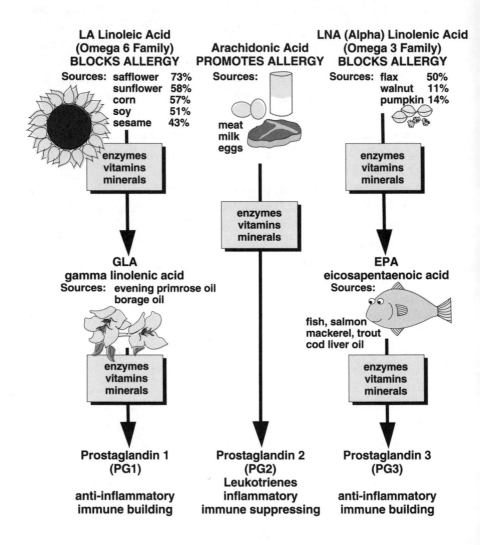

LA Linoleic Acid (Omega 6 Family) BLOCKS ALLERGY	Arachidonic Acid PROMOTES ALLERGY	LNA (Alpha) Linolenic Acid (Omega 3 Family) BLOCKS ALLERGY

Sources: safflower 73%, sunflower 58%, corn 57%, soy 51%, sesame 43%

Sources: meat, milk, eggs

Sources: flax 50%, walnut 11%, pumpkin 14%

enzymes vitamins minerals

GLA
gamma linolenic acid
Sources: evening primrose oil, borage oil

EPA
eicosapentaenoic acid
Sources: fish, salmon, mackerel, trout, cod liver oil

Prostaglandin 1 (PG1)	Prostaglandin 2 (PG2) Leukotrienes	Prostaglandin 3 (PG3)
anti-inflammatory immune building	inflammatory immune suppressing	anti-inflammatory immune building

Figure 6. Important Pathways

any of these factors are missing, the conversion cannot take place. One necessary and important enzyme is called Delta 6 desaturase. It can be inactivated by several common factors, including drugs such as cortisone, alcohol, tobacco, excess saturated fat in the diet and heated fats such as the fats in fried food. When these factors are present, Delta 6 desaturase cannot convert beneficial oils into anti-inflammatory prostaglandins. Although inflammation is a normal and necessary part of the healing reaction, wild, unchecked inflammation is destructive and tissue damaging. This is attested to by the millions of dollars spent every year on anti-inflammatory drugs.

What people do not understand is that the body produces its own anti-inflammatory substances in the form of prostaglandins. All it needs is the necessary raw materials from foods with which to work.

In order to make good choices, it is essential to learn about the proper oils and how to obtain them. You are probably familiar with the fact that white sugar is a refined product. Refined sugar is stripped of its nutrients with only the carbohydrates left. White flour is also a nutrient-poor, refined product. Unfortunately, it is no different for oils. The safflower oil sitting on the supermarket shelf has been refined and the LA it contained has been virtually destroyed in the manufacturing process.

When oil is refined several toxic products are formed including trans-fatty acids. Fats and oils are very sensitive to light, heat and oxygen. You cannot heat or cook any kind of oil without producing toxic by-products. Commercial oils of safflower, corn and sunflower have been heated to temperatures of 464 to 518 degrees F for 30 to 60 minutes, forming trans-fatty acids.

The very molecules of the oil have been denatured. They have been forced into a new, unnatural shape, becoming straight, while the normal shape is curved or horseshoe-shaped. The problem is that these abnormal, straightened molecules do not fit into the biological membranes of the cells in the same way as the horseshoe-shaped molecules. It is like trying to put the wrong piece in a jigsaw puzzle: it just doesn't fit. The molecules of the refined oil only partially fit the cell membranes. They take up the space, but can't do the work. The worst damaging effect is that trans-fatty acids block out natural healthful fat so that it cannot function. Trans-fatty acids get incorporated into many tissues, including the heart, whose normal fuel is fatty acids.

Since enzymes break down the trans-fatty acids more slowly than the natural horseshoe-shaped fatty acids, impaired function may result.

Another destructive aspect of trans-fatty acids is that, while residing in unsaturated fat, they act more like saturated fat. Trans-fatty acids are sticky and cause blood cells to clump together. They can cause fatty deposits in blood vessels by altering cholesterol metabolism. Trans-fatty acids are powerful immune-system inhibitors that block enzymes, which help the production of prostaglandins. Since they displace natural fats at the cell membrane, they reduce oxygen supply to the cell. On the other hand, natural fats attract oxygen, which is their normal physiological function.

The nervous system consists primarily of fat tissue. Trans-fatty acids help promote degeneration of nerves. Trans-fatty acids can trigger the release of inflammatory arachidonic acid products from cells. Worst of all, Trans-fatty acids disrupt the vital activities of the natural fats and create a deficiency of the fatty acids essential for life: LA and LNA.

There is even more bad news. Trans-fatty acids are found in nearly all packaged and processed foods. If the package says hydrogenated or partially hydrogenated vegetable oil, it contains trans-fatty acids. The average intake of trans-fatty acids is about twelve grams per day, which is nearly twice as much as all the other food additives put together.

Major sources of trans-fatty acids are margarine, vegetable oil and shortening. Stick margarine averages 31% trans-fatty acids, but can be as high as 47%. Vegetable oil shortenings may contain over 37% trans-fatty acids. In contrast, European oils cannot contain more than 1% trans-fatty acids, and the Dutch government has banned the sale of margarine containing trans-fatty acids.

Margarine is simply not the healthful product that the public has been led to believe. In addition to trans-fatty acids, it contains dozens of other toxic compounds produced by the hydrogenation process and by the heat, light and oxygen that its oils are exposed to in the refining process. Recent studies show that margarine may actually raise blood cholesterol levels.

The amounts of essential fatty acids that margarine contains have been greatly reduced by the refining process. Udo Erasmus, author of *Fats and Oils* states "Margarines, the way they are now manufactured, are dangerous to health, especially when consumed to excess."

Studies show that it takes over seven weeks to remove half of the trans-fatty acids from the heart. Trans-fatty acids can be removed by increasing consumption of LNA, found in flaxseed oil, while simultaneously decreasing intake of products containing trans-fatty acids.

Products that Contain Trans-fatty Acids

Percentage of Trans-fatty Acids (high to low)	Product
30-40%	Candies, cookies, frostings
37%	French fries
24-34%	Corn chips
33% (up to)	Doughnuts and pastries
20-30%	Crackers
24% (up to)	Bread and rolls
13%	Salad oil

In addition to the oils already mentioned, beneficial foods that can be used to supplement the diet are evening primrose oil and microalgae. Evening primrose oil contains gamma-linoleic acid (GLA). It is normally formed from LA. It follows the anti-inflammatory PG1 pathway. Microalgae provide the main sources of eicosapentaenoic acid (EPA); they are the source of the EPA found in fish. EPA is normally formed from LNA. EPA displaces arachidonic acid, keeping blood free flowing. It also has anti-inflammatory properties. Flaxseed, hempseed, and walnut oils are also sources of LNA, but some individuals need a direct source of EPA, such as microalgae.

An important point to remember is that LA and LNA are natural fats designed to do life-supporting work in the body. Trans-fatty acids are the by-products in man-made processed foods. Trans-fatty acids are foreign to, and cannot be beneficially used by, the body.

Another major problem with fats that have been heated to high temperatures, either in the refining process or by frying, is the formation of free radicals. Simply speaking, free radicals are highly reactive molecules which move with lightning speed through the body. They are a primary cause of cellular damage, old age skin spots and wrinkling of the skin. Free radicals damage the outer membranes of the cells so that they cannot hold tightly together, causing the skin to sag or wrinkle. In severe damage, the cells die and rise to the skin surface, forming the brown skin spots we see in elderly people. High fat diets and chemical toxins encourage the process of cellular damage by free radicals.

Exposing the body to external sources of radiation can also form these highly reactive molecules.

Cells can be protected from free radical damage by avoiding both internal and external causes of free radical formation. Common sources of free radicals include refined and rancid fats, fried food, chemical pollutants and radiation.

Essential fatty acid deficiency is probably the most common, but least recognized, nutritional deficiency. This deficiency leads to immune system breakdown setting the stage for allergy. People experiencing fatty acid deficiency are prone to allergies, sinus problems, hay fever, asthma, psoriasis, eczema, premenstrual syndrome and other conditions.

Symptoms of Essential Fatty Acid Deficiency
Bleeding gums
Dry, flaky skin
Dry, brittle or oily hair
Brittle nails
Cold hands and feet
Excess ear wax
Lowered resistance to infection
Hair loss

The immune system cannot function well without essential fatty acids. In fact, it has been shown that cells and organs will degenerate if essential fatty acids are not supplied by the diet. Children are especially dependent upon LA and LNA for brain development. Besides being caused by direct deficiency in the diet, essential fatty acid deficiency can be created by common dietary practices such as:

1. Chronic intake of alcohol.
2. High intake of refined sugar.
3. Excess intake of saturated fat.
4. Intake of hydrogenated, partially hydrogenated or deep-fried fats.
5. Smoking.
6. Use of drugs such as cortisone, or the overuse of antibiotics.

Natural Foods that Contain Essential Fatty Acids
Avocado
Beans
Hempseed
Flaxseed
Green leafy vegetables
Nuts (raw, unsalted)
Pumpkin seeds (raw, unsalted)
Sesame seeds
Sunflower seeds

Canola oil is the most unsaturated oil available on the market, and for this reason has been promoted as being healthful. Used in its unrefined form, this may be true. However, most canola available to the public is refined and therefore subject to forming the same toxic substances as other oils namely, Trans-fatty acids and free radicals.

Another concern with canola has been its content of erucic acid. Through laboratory studies done with canola, erucic acid was thought to cause fatty degeneration of the heart, kidney, adrenals and thyroid of rats. Based on this assumption, new varieties of low erucic acid rapeseed were bred and government standards limited the erucic acid content of canola to 5% or less.

According to Udo Erasmus, author of *Fats That Heal, Fats That Kill*, it now appears that other oils such as sunflower that contains no erucic acid will cause the same degenerative changes in rats as canola.

Evidently, rats do not metabolize fats and oils well, and there are indications that rat metabolism in this respect may differ substantially from human fat metabolism. More recent findings indicate that canola oil will not cause the same problems in human hearts as in rat hearts. Consequently, it appears that the erucic acid content of canola is not so toxic as once believed.

Cottonseed oil is often used in margarine and mayonnaise. However, since cotton is not a food crop, chemicals banned for use on food crops are not banned for cotton. Highly toxic chemicals such as paraquat and arsenic have been used on cotton crops. Cottonseed oil may contain residues of these toxic chemicals and therefore cannot be recommended. Cottonseed oil contains cyclopropene fatty acid, which has known toxic effects on the liver and gall bladder. In addition to margarine and mayonnaise, cottonseed oil often appears in crackers, salad dressing, potato chips and other chips, and baking mixes.

Using Healthful Oils

While the various metabolic pathways of fats and oils may seem complicated to the person unfamiliar with biochemistry, making use of the information about oils is fairly simple. There are only a few key points that a person must know in order to get the good elements from fats and oils and eliminate the harmful ones.

Using Healthful Fats and Oils - Simplified

• First, eliminate all fried foods. The high heat of frying alters the oil, producing trans-fatty acids, free radicals and other toxic products.
• Second, use only cold-pressed oil found in dark bottles in the refrigerated portion of the health food store. Make your own salad dressings and mayonnaise with these oils. Include flaxseed or hempseed oils in your diet. If you purchase a product that already has oil added to it, you can almost be sure the oil is refined, toxic and nutrient deficient.
• Third, if you sauté or stir-fry vegetables such, use only a small quantity, one tablespoon or less, of butter or extra virgin olive oil.

172

These are the only two fats that should ever be heated, as they are more stable and produce the least toxic substances. Adding chopped onions or garlic to the fat in the pan helps protect the fat from oxidation and produces even less toxic elements. Better yet, substitute a small amount of broth or water for oil when preparing a dish that calls for sautéing or stir-frying.

- Fourth, use butter rather than margarine. Since butter is a saturated fat, it should be used in small quantities. However, it is more digestible than margarine and contains less chemicals and toxic products.
- Fifth, add ground up flaxseed or hempseed to cereals and salads. A coffee grinder will grind a small amount for immediate use. Never store these ground seeds and never cook with flaxseed or hempseed oils, as they become toxic when heated.
- Sixth, get a book that tells you how much fat, in grams, you are eating each day. Keep track of this for one week. The amount of fat should not exceed 20% of the calories eaten. That would be 40 grams on a 2,000-calorie diet. Systematically cut fat down to this level, eliminating the sources of refined oils and adding in unrefined oils.

Unrefined Oils - Good sources of LA

Safflower	73% linoleic
Sunflower	58% linoleic
Corn	57% linoleic
Soy	51% linoleic

Unrefined Oils - Good sources of LNA

Flaxseed oil	50% linolenic
Poppy seed oil	30% linolenic
Hempseed oil	20% linolenic
Pumpkin seed oil	15% linolenic
Walnut oil	11% linolenic
Soybean oil	7% linolenic

Good sources of LNA are less common. The unrefined oils of flaxseed or hempseed contains some LA as well, making them the most important oils you can add to your diet.

Tasty Ways to Use Oils

Whenever we start to use new products in new ways, there can be stumbling blocks. It takes time, effort and thought to incorporate new ideas in the kitchen. A few key recipes are included here in order to help you get started using the essential oils that are beneficial, and to show you how easy it can be to use seeds and nuts. All the recipes are easy, quick to prepare and very tasty.

Instant Breakfast

This recipe contains the essential oils that the body can quickly burn for energy, that are necessary for brain growth and function and that help normalize cholesterol. It is also high in organic trace minerals and calcium. Ounce for ounce, sesame seeds contain more calcium than milk.

All seeds used are raw, unsalted.
Mix together and soak in 3/4 cup of pure water for 24 hours:
1 tbsp. pumpkin seeds
1 tbsp. sesame seeds
1 tbsp. flaxseed or hempseed
2 tbsp. almonds
1 tbsp. sunflower seeds
Pour into blender and liquefy while adding 1 cup of water. Add two to three tsp. raw, unpasteurized honey. Add 1 to 11/2 cups of frozen or fresh berries, cherries, or banana. Makes two large glasses.

Millet Cereal with Pureed Pears

This cereal is chewy and tasty as is, but a variation can be made by creaming it in the blender. This will have a texture that is more familiar to children. To cream cereal, put about 1/2 cup cooked grain in the blender and add hot water slowly while blending until the desired consistency is reached.

Soak 1 cup of organic millet in 2 cups of water for 12 hours.

When you are ready for bed, pour the grain into a casserole dish or crock-pot. Bake all night in the oven or cook in a crock-pot at the lowest setting (120° to 150° F). When you get up in the morning, the cereal is hot and ready to eat.

For topping, puree 1 can unsweetened pears in the blender and spoon over cereal. Cereal may also be topped with pureed peaches or with unpasteurized honey, molasses, cinnamon, chopped dried fruits, raisins, dates, warm unsweetened apple juice, and pure maple syrup or seed and nut milk.

Millet cereal is the most digestible grain and the least likely grain to create food reactions. Cereal made in the above manner contains fiber, B vitamins, minerals and a small amount of essential fatty acids. Other variations of the above recipe may be made by using other types of grain such as barley or oats.

Seed and Nut Milk Basic Recipe
½ cup raw almonds
¼ cup sesame seeds

Soak in 2 cups of pure water for 24 hours. Pour into blender and blend as you add enough water to fill the blender. Add unpasteurized honey to taste, (approximately 1 tablespoon) Add 1 teaspoon vanilla, or to taste. Pour through strainer.

Nut milk will keep in the refrigerator approximately three days. Store in a dark bottle if possible. This nut milk is high in calcium, and contains essential oils and trace minerals in a form easily utilized by the body. Any raw nuts can be used to make nut milk. However, sesame seeds and almonds are highest in calcium. Flaxseed or hempseed can also be added to this recipe in order to raise the content of LNA. Nut milk may be used over cereal, over berries or in recipes, or it may be drunk from a glass.

Commercial Mayonnaise

Commercial mayonnaise is often made from cottonseed oil or other vegetable oils that have been refined at high temperatures and exposed to light and oxygen, creating many toxic by-products including Trans-fatty acids. Through such treatment, the essential fatty acids, LA and LNA, have been degraded. Many health authorities simply advise against eating mayonnaise at all. However, it is easy to make mayonnaise, a healthful product, which contributes essential nutrients to your diet, whether you make a sandwich to take to school or a dip to eat with vegetables. You must remember, however, that even good quality mayonnaise is nearly 100% fat and should be used in small quantities.

Homemade Mayonnaise

Use oil labeled unrefined or cold-pressed, sold in a dark bottle in the refrigerator of the health food store. This mixture tastes like regular mayonnaise, but will be slightly cream-colored. For lighter color, eliminate the flax or hemp oil and use 1 cup of the safflower only.

1 fresh free range egg
5 tsp. fresh lemon juice
2 tsp. Dijon mustard
½ tsp. sea salt (optional)
Dash of Tabasco sauce
1 cup combination of unrefined oil (¾ cup safflower, sunflower or walnut oil and ¼ cup flaxseed or hempseed oil)

Add egg, juice, mustard, salt and Tabasco to blender and blend for 5 seconds until mixed. Add oil slowly in a thin stream until thickened mayonnaise texture is achieved. Store mayonnaise in the refrigerator for up to two weeks.

Whipped Butter

Use one part butter to one part flaxseed or hempseed oil. Blend softened butter and oil in blender. Store in the refrigerator up to three days. This recipe helps cut down the amount of saturated fat of the butter while supplying the essential oils necessary for health. This butter must not be used in cooking.

Salad Dressing - Basic Recipe

¼ cup unrefined oil (combination of safflower, sunflower, walnut, flaxseed, or hempseed oils)
2 cloves fresh garlic, minced
¼ cup fresh lemon juice
Pinch of sea salt, if desired

Any other seasoning you wish to add such as fresh herbs, onion, etc. or a packet of salad seasonings obtained from your health food store. Blend together in blender. Store in refrigerator.

Avocado Dressing

1 medium avocado, ripe
2 cloves garlic, minced
2 rounded tbsp. chopped onions
¼ cup of unrefined oil
sea salt, to taste

Blend in blender until smooth. Serve on salad immediately.

Easy Caesar Dressing

This recipe can be made ahead and stored in a covered, dark container in the refrigerator. It is best when made a day ahead of use.

½ cup unrefined oil (a mixture of safflower oil, and walnut oil, flaxseed, or hempseed oil is good)
1 fresh free range egg
1 tbsp. Worcestershire sauce
⅓ cup fresh lemon juice
2 cloves garlic, coarsely chopped
pinch of sea salt
¼ tsp. freshly ground pepper
½ cup freshly grated Parmesan cheese
Optional ingredient: can of anchovies

Blend all ingredients until smooth.

Vegetable Dip - Children Can Become Vegetable Lovers

Children like small chunks of raw vegetables that they can dip. Serve vegetables to children an hour before dinner. While they are dipping, you can prepare the rest of the meal in peace.

Cut up raw vegetables. Experiment with new vegetables and new shapes such as carrot curls, carved animals from turnips, cucumbers and fresh broccoli.

Use avocado dressing for dip, or make a dip using the mayonnaise recipe. Take equal quantities of mayonnaise and low or non-fat yogurt as a base. Mix in seasonings, such as curry, onion, garlic or whatever your children enjoy.

Vegetable Juice

Another pre-dinner idea is to juice the vegetables. Use carrots for a base. Good proportions are 80% carrot juice and 20% green vegetables such as: celery, parsley, watercress, broccoli, and cabbage. If juice seems bitter, add one apple and serve. Most children will enjoy this juice if served fresh and if greens are held to a minimum at first. Then add greater quantities of greens as they get used to the idea of drinking the vegetables. Many juice books are available at health food stores for extra ideas.

15

Six Unsuspected Allergic Conditions in Children

Krista's Success Story as Told by Her Mother

Roughly one year ago, 7-year-old Krista was suffering from the effects of numerous food allergies. Today she is able to enjoy a varied diet, which includes most of the foods that she previously could not tolerate.

After reading Dr. Bateson-Koch's book, *Allergies: Disease in Disguise*, I realized that Dr. Bateson-Koch had the key to solving Krista's allergy problems. So, in June, Krista and I made the 600-mile trip to Dr. Bateson-Koch's office.

Since birth, Krista had been living with pain in her digestive system; there were many nights when she did not sleep at all. She would lie on the couch while I rubbed her back and stomach to try to give her some comfort. She had frequent eye infections and her eyes would puff up and discharge as a reaction to some foods. As a baby, she had frequent ear infections. She was always small for her age, and very underweight. While Krista understood everything she was told, her speech was limited mostly to single words. On better days, she sometimes used three or four word sentences. Other days, she would communicate by using single words or pointing and saying "uh, uh".

Krista's family medical doctor was unable to offer any advice at all with her allergy problems. So after quite a lot of research, I was very pleased to find Dr. Bateson-Koch's book and even happier to meet the doctor in person.

After a morning of testing, examination, and chiropractic adjustments, Dr. Bateson-Koch was able to identify the underlying conditions causing Krista's food reactions and devise a program of supplements to boost her immune system back to a healthy state.

One of the immediate results of the treatments was that Krista was able to fall asleep and sleep peacefully through the whole night. Previously, she often couldn't sleep until the early hours of the morning because her digestion was bothering her. Another immediate result was that her moods became more even.

We attended Dr. Bateson-Koch's clinic for several days in order for Dr. Bateson-Koch to follow up and be sure the supplements were taking effect, and to have chiropractic adjustments. Not having been treated by a chiropractor before, I was amazed at the effectiveness of the adjustments.

After returning home, Krista had weekly chiropractic adjustments from a local chiropractor. She also followed the program of nutritional supplements and diet that Dr. Bateson-Koch had outlined.

In August, we again made the long trip to Dr. Bateson-Koch's office for a check-up. Krista was improved to the point where some of her problem foods could be added back into her diet. Some of the vitamin supplements were continued, as well as plant enzymes to aid digestion.

At the next follow up appointment with Dr. Bateson-Koch in November, Krista had no reaction to her problem foods when tested. Since then, eating has been much more enjoyable for her because she is now able to eat the same foods as the rest of the family. She no longer has stomach pains; she is growing well, sleeping well, and her speech is improving. The eye and ear infections are gone. This winter is the first that Krista has not been sick, even for a single day.

Common Childhood Conditions

Six very common childhood conditions are often manifestations of allergy and intolerance, but they are seldom treated as allergic problems. Usually unsuspected as allergic in nature, these conditions are colic in infants, ear infections, bed-wetting, eczema, asthma, and hyperactivity.

Colic

Colic is so common that newborn babies are almost expected to have it. However, James C. Breneman, MD considers it to be "a definite manifestation of intolerance, much of which is allergic." In this condition, and especially in infants whose entire diet is milk, cow's milk is overwhelmingly the leading allergen. A baby who is breast-fed may still develop an allergy to cow's milk if the mother ingests milk, cheese, yogurt or other dairy products.

Cow's milk proteins in the form of immune complexes can be transmitted to a baby through breast milk, causing sensitization in the infant. Intestinal biopsies have been performed on infants with colic after they were fed cow's milk for seven days. Increased IgE levels, indicating allergy, have been found in the cells of the biopsy samples.

Breast milk is in the raw state. It has not been cooked or heated, so it is a very enzyme-dense product. The enzymes contained in breast milk help the baby digest the milk, taking stress off its immature digestive tract. Infant formulas contain no enzymes and force the infant's digestive organs to do all the work. Cow's milk formula is higher in protein and fat than breast milk, giving the baby's digestive tract even more of a workout. If the baby's digestive tract is unable to produce sufficient enzymes to digest the cow's milk formula, colic will result. Since the baby's immature digestive tract is naturally more permeable than an older child's, it allows easier absorption of partially digested protein particles, leading to allergy.

Colic is easily remedied in a baby. In the breast-fed baby, the mother should eliminate all sources of dairy products from her diet. The baby should be given nutritional plant enzymes each time it is fed. For the formula-fed infant, the formulas should be rotated every four to five days from soy formula, to goat's milk formula and the various other formulas that can be found. Each time the baby is fed, nutritional plant enzymes should be supplemented.

Common Symptoms of Food Allergy in a Baby

Unfortunately, colic is only one symptom of food allergy in a baby. Here is a list of others.

Bloodshot eyes	Hives or welts
Bronchitis	Irritability
Chronic cough	Loose bowels
Cold sores	Nasal stuffiness, sniffling,

Colic	snorting, sneezing
Diaper rash, redness at anus	Nose rubbing
or on cheeks	Rashes
Eczema	Tiny broken blood vessels
Frequent colds	under the skin
Fussy eater	Wheezing

It is ironic that we feed the most allergenic food known to man to our babies and children. B-lactoglobulin, a substance found in cow's milk, but not in human milk, is foreign to the baby's digestive tract. Newborn babies have increased gastrointestinal permeability to B-lactoglobulin, probably because of a lack of enzymes to digest it. Casein is another of the most allergenic proteins in milk.

Allergy to milk creates gastrointestinal bleeding, which leads to iron-deficiency anemia in infants, due to a loss of blood in the stool. If the blood comes from high up in the intestinal tract, it will appear as dark or black and is not readily recognized. This blood loss can go undetected for long periods resulting in iron deficiency in the child. Other diseases that have been associated with milk include celiac disease, chronic diarrhea, various gastroenteropathies, pulmonary manifestations and fibrosis.

Amy's Success Story

Amy was only ten months old when her mother brought her to my office. She was showing obvious signs of food allergy and had eczema. Her mother was breast feeding her, as Amy could not tolerate other forms of food. She was not even doing well on the breast milk. She had frequent colic and a rash on her arms and legs. Examination of the infant showed that she was intolerant to all milk, including breast milk. She reacted strongly to tobacco smoke and sugar. There was under-functioning of the pancreas, liver and kidneys.

Treatment consisted of chiropractic adjustments to help align and balance the body. Amy was to have concentrated plant enzymes each time she ate and a nutritional supplement daily. Her mother was told to refrain from all dairy products, as allergenic particles from milk can be present in the breast milk. She was told to continue breast-feeding and not to introduce new foods for the time being.

Over the next few weeks, the eczema and stomach distress disappeared. After eight weeks, the mother was successfully able to introduce some fruits and vegetables into the diet. Amy continued to improve, and eight months after beginning treatment she was able to tolerate all food groups without a return of symptoms. Her pancreas, liver and kidneys tested normal. One and a half years later, Amy had had no recurrence of symptoms and was a healthy, normal youngster.

Ear Infection - Childhood's Most Common Illness

Each year 30 million children in the United States are treated for middle ear infections reflecting a 300% increase in the last twenty years.

Middle ear infection is the number one condition for doctor visits by children under the age of 15. Current estimates are that 65% of children will have at least one ear infection before the age of one and 90% will have at least one ear infection before the age of three. Middle ear infection is the most common reason for surgery in children and it is the leading cause of deafness in children.

Understanding Ear Infection

The structure of a young child's ear is different than an adult's ear. In a child, the immature Eustachian tube is shorter and more horizontal than in an adult. As a child grows, a characteristic downward curve develops until, at maturity, there is a pronounced downward angle that has developed. This allows fluids to drain more readily and accounts for why some children seem to outgrow their symptoms as they get older. However, even when children appear to outgrow their symptoms, the underlying or precipitating mechanism, which originally produced the ear problem, may still be in place, often resulting in new symptoms appearing somewhere else in the child's body.

Eustachian Tube Dysfunction

The Eustachian tube leads from the middle ear to the area in back of the nose and throat. This tube performs two vital functions. It keeps the air pressure equal on both sides of the eardrum and allows excess fluid to drain away from the ear. The pop you hear when yawning or swallowing is the Eustachian tube equalizing the air pressure in the middle ear.

When there is obstruction of the Eustachian tube, ear fluid cannot drain properly, often resulting in fluid build-up in the middle ear and the possibility of an infection starting. When infections originate in the throat, nasal areas or tonsils, the pathogenic bacteria often migrate up the Eustachian tube to the middle ear. Common causes for Eustachian tube obstruction are a complication of colds and flu, allergic or non-allergic inflammation of the membranes of the nose and surrounding tissues, acute or chronic sinusitis and enlargement of the adenoids.

Is it Infection or Inflammation?

Ear symptoms do not always mean ear infection. Confusion arises when both parents and health care professionals may mistake ear inflammation with ear infection (presence of bacterial or viral organisms). Inflammation that produces redness, swelling, and heat of the middle ear without infection is called Otitis media

Acute Otitis media means inflammation of the middle ear with signs of infection. This last category accounts for the vast majority of ear symptoms. However, the escalation in numbers of recurrent ear infections in recent years has prompted another term for ear infection to evolve - chronic Otitis media. Since all ear disorders are not necessarily infection, the term middle ear syndrome is probably more descriptive.

It is usually the fluid build-up of the middle ear that causes pain. Normally the middle ear is filled with air, but as fluid accumulates and pushes on the inside of the eardrum, pain develops. Sometimes the pressure in the middle ear may build up to a point where the eardrum bursts, which results in fluid or pus and blood drainage from the ear.

Conventional Treatment

Antibiotics are the mainstays of conventional treatment for middle ear infections. An estimated 25 million prescriptions (over one billion individual doses) for antibiotics are written for children with ear infection each year in the United States. Antibiotics are commonly prescribed for either five or ten day courses. Analgesics to relieve pain and reduce fever may also be used. If the child has three or more episodes of acute Otitis media within six months, or suffers a serious hearing loss, surgery is usually recommended.

A surgery called *myringotomy* with implantation of ear tubes is usually performed under general anesthesia, and is the most common operation performed on children today. The surgeon places tiny plastic tubes in the ears to allow drainage from the middle ear to the outer ear canal. This forms a sort of by-pass for the Eustachian tube providing air ventilation for the middle ear. The tubes stay in place from three to eighteen months, with six months being average, before they are extruded into the ear canal. In some cases, the surgical procedure must be repeated two or three times. Scarring of the tympanic membrane (eardrum) and loss of hearing are side effects of tympanostomy. At best, tympanostomy is a symptomatic treatment.

Are Antibiotics Effective?

Although antibiotics are the standard treatment, they provide only temporary, symptomatic relief and no protection against recurring episodes.

A recent study done on the effectiveness of antibiotics for middle ear infection demonstrated that after treatment with amoxicillin, 69% of the children still had Otitis media (middle ear inflammation). Another study showed that amoxicillin administration conferred no more protection against acute episodes than a placebo.

Numerous studies show that antibiotics do not prevent the reoccurrence of ear infection. According to David S. Hurst, MD, after twenty-five years of practice as an ear, nose and throat surgeon, "Conventional therapy with antibiotics has proven to be ineffective, yet is still maintained in the current management paradigm." He goes on to state, "The current algorithm is still to treat children 1-3 years old who present with an acute infection with antibiotics until they resolve. Although by definition Otitis media with effusion is fluid with no signs of infection, it is advised that Otitis media with effusion be treated with antibiotics until the fluid resolves." Dr.

Hurst then cites twenty-eight studies regarding the use of antibiotics for chromic Otitis media. All of these studies conclude that antibiotics are no more effective than a placebo in achieving resolution of the fluid in the ears.

Dr. Michael Schmidt reports, "There are a substantial number of children who continue to have middle ear infection despite repeated antibiotic therapy. In many cases (up to 75%), the fluid contains no bacteria."

Even though antibiotics and ear tubes are routine treatment for ear infections, they are not without controversy within the medical community. An understanding as to when these therapies may be appropriate as well as inappropriate and the advantages and disadvantages of the therapies are extremely important considerations.

Considerations For Antibiotic Use

1. Antibiotics help to resolve bacterial infection in the middle ear and may reduce the risk of more serious spread of infection.
2. Use of antibiotics reduces the risk of pain, after 2-7 days, by 40%.
3. Use of an antibiotic may prevent infection from developing in the other ear.

Considerations Against Antibiotic Use

1. Antibiotics have side effects which may produce vomiting, diarrhea, skin rash or allergic reactions. Some antibiotics cause a thinning of the lining of the intestinal tract, producing inflammation and poor absorption of vitamins, minerals, and fats.
2. Recent studies indicate that only one child in seven children with ear infection will benefit from antibiotic use.
3. Frequent use of antibiotics allows bacteria to develop resistance to the drugs. Currently, bacterial resistance to antibiotics is developing faster than the drug companies can produce new antibiotics.
4. Antibiotics destroy healthy intestinal bacteria. Researchers are now reporting that friendly bacterial flora is estimated to comprise up to 80% of the child's immune system. Beneficial colon bacteria perform vital functions which range from manufacturing vitamins to controlling the growth of pathological organisms.

5. Some antibiotics inhibit activity of white blood cells, and inhibit antibody production.
6. A 1991 study demonstrated that children with earaches, who received antibiotics, especially in the first few days of illness, were much more likely to develop recurrent ear problems than those in whom treatment was delayed.
7. When antibiotics are effective, they give temporary resolution and do not address predisposing conditions, which are left to perpetuate recurring episodes of ear infection.

Allergy in the Ears

Is there evidence that allergens can produce changes in the middle ear? In his book, *Childhood Ear Infections*, Dr. Michael A. Schmidt makes the statement, "Allergens can cause direct changes within the middle ear and Eustachian tube." Dr. Schmidt cites as an example that Dr. Robert O'Conner and his colleagues observed significant and rapid pressure changes take place in the middle ear of children when their nasal passages were exposed to allergens. In other studies, allergens have been found capable of causing obstruction of the Eustachian tube for up to fourteen days.

For over fifty years, allergy has been shown to play a role in middle ear syndrome. Doctors are increasingly speaking out and identifying the ear as the target organ for underlying allergies, especially food allergies. In his book, Childhood Illness and the Allergy Connection, Zoltan Rona, MD, makes the statement; "Allergies to milk and other common foods and the frequent and indiscriminate use of prescription antibiotics are at the root of most infections in children, especially middle-ear infections." This is a profound statement and many doctors who take this approach to middle ear dysfunction are finding it to be true by their often-dramatic clinical results.

Dr. George Shambaugh, Professor Emeritus of Otolaryngology at Northwestern University stated in an address in 1982,

Although allergies in children are often hard to identify by the usual allergy scratch tests, I've found that a program of allergic management with attention to hidden or delayed-in-onset food allergy helps me manage recurrent ear problems in children. Moreover, my results with allergy management are far better than those obtained by putting children on prolonged courses of antibiotics, and relying on tubes to clear up the condition.

A study of 512 children with allergy and middle ear infection conducted by Dr. John P. McGovern demonstrated that when careful allergy management was followed, the results with 97% of the children ranged from good to excellent. A major factor of fluid accumulation in the middle ear is the blockage of the Eustachian tube, which normally drains fluids away from the ear.

Bruce A. Epstein, MD, writes "Nasal allergies may cause the child to have chronic nasal congestion and swelling of tissue lining the Eustachian tube."

Clinical studies show that allergy plays a major role in middle ear dysfunction. A study of 448 patients with middle ear infection revealed that 57% had asthma, a confirmed allergic problem, while 95% had allergic rhinitis (inflammation of the nose), and 16% had dermatitis (rash). Another study confirmed that half of the children in the study with allergic disease also had middle ear dysfunction. Still other studies reveal that both IgE and IgG antibodies against specific foods have been isolated in the serum and the middle ear fluids of Otitis susceptible children. Of these antibodies, the one for milk is the most common, followed by egg, and then wheat.

Various other studies reveal that factors which promote Eustachian tube dysfunction leading to Otitis media include: allergic reactions, infectious inflammation, persistent pathogenic bacteria and their components, and viruses. In their 1965 article, "Secretory Otitis media in allergic infants and children," which appeared in *Southern Medical Journal,* 1965, Fernandez and McGovern suggested allergic mechanism as the major cause of chronic Otitis media as well as a predisposing factor in as many as 85% of children with acute Otitis.

Protection for Ear Infection

New studies suggest that breast-feeding of infants has a protective effect against infections of the middle ear. In 256 infants, the incidence of Otitis media was inversely associated with the duration of breast-feeding. In other words, the longer the infant was breast-fed, the fewer middle ear infections. A Boston study of 692 children also indicated that "Breast feeding was associated significantly with decreased risk of recurrent acute Otitis media."

Why would breast-feed make such a difference? There are several explanations:

1. Allergy to one or more components in cow's or formula milk. It is well known that swelling of tissues is an effect of allergy. In this case the mucosa of the Eustachian tube swells, closing the opening from the nasopharynx to the middle ear. Once the Eustachian tube is blocked, fluid begins to collect in the middle ear, often resulting in infection.

2. Breast milk conveys immunological factors to the infant, which help prevent bacterial and viral infections. It contains immunoglobulins and various types of white blood cells. Breast milk prevents the attachment of Pneumococci and Haemophilus influenza (pneumonia and flu-causing bacteria) to epithelial cells.

3. Breast milk is in the raw, uncooked state, which means that it contains natural enzymes to aid in its digestion, requiring little digestive effort on the part of the infant.

   Cow's milk and infant formulas have been heat-treated through pasteurization at temperatures high enough to kill all the enzymes. In order to digest this milk, the infant must supply all of the enzymes from its own digestive fluids. If its immature digestive tract cannot supply all the needed enzymes, incomplete digestion takes place. Partially digested protein particles can now pass through the intestinal lining and into the general circulation, causing an allergic response. The fact that IgE and IgG antibodies have been isolated in inner ear fluids indicates the ear is a site for the allergic reaction. Cow's milk and infant formulas are much higher in protein content than breast milk, putting an additional load on the infant's digestive tract and allowing more potential for incompletely digested protein to enter the general circulation.

4. Antibiotics used to treat middle ear infection may lead to candidiasis.

   Clinical studies show that Candida is usually present in the middle ear after one or two episodes of middle ear infection. A baby can also be born with this condition if the mother has candidiasis. This chronic infection keeps the ear in a weakened condition of lowered immunity and may allow new infections of bacteria to occur.

Dr. C. Oran Truss was among the first to raise the alarm that Candida albicans was capable of infecting so many parts of the body and creating a multitude of symptoms. His 1983 book, *The Missing Diagnosis*, linked Candida to allergies and many other conditions.

Dr. Truss was probably the first to link Candida albicans to recurrent ear infections. Referring to systemic candidiasis, he explains, "And finally, all of the familiar manifestations of allergy are common. Once these membranes of the respiratory tract become inflamed by their allergic response to yeast products, infections begin to occur with great regularity at random sites from the nose to the lungs. Depending upon location, the infection is known as a cold, sinus infection, sore throat, Otitis (ear), bronchitis, or pneumonia."

William G. Crook, MD, in his best selling book, *The Yeast Connection*, continues this line of exploration citing his own experiences as a pediatrician and those of others. While acknowledging that Candida may be one of several factors involved in chronic ear problems, he concludes, "Moreover, my own experience in using nystatin and a special diet in a limited number of children with recurrent ear problems makes me feel that an anti-candida treatment program in these children is appropriate."

More recently (January, 2000) Dr. Crook has written *Nature's Own Candida Cure* in which he refers to health problems in children including recurrent ear disorders; "These problems are increasing in frequency and current methods of management appear to be ineffective. These problems are often yeast-related."

The greatest mistake in the treatment and management of ear infection is the view taken by most doctors that it is a localized problem with treatment directed at the ear only. Even the numerous failures of this approach has not changed the conventional recommendations for treatment, antibiotics and surgery. Evidence is mounting to show that the ear is the secondary effect of conditions that have developed elsewhere in the body. Although it is becoming apparent that treatment of the ear alone is not adequate, many doctors have, nevertheless, failed to recognize other common factors within the body that can trigger symptoms in the middle ear and perpetuate them.

How to Help Your Child Recover

Prevention is the most important part of any health program, but it is never too late to begin. Regardless of how many antibiotics and tubal surgeries that your child may have experienced, there is still much you can do to prevent further episodes. Developed over 30 years of clinical experience, the following program has proven to be an effective, natural method to resolve childhood ear infections.

1. Supplement with probiotics (friendly intestinal bacteria) to reculture the colon. Good quality products are kept in the refrigerated portion of the health food store. They come in powder or capsule form. For very young children, the powder form is best or capsules may be opened and mixed with a small amount of food. Probiotics should be taken daily for approximately three months. While dosage depends on body weight, approximately one teaspoon a day is a good guide.

2. Include grapefruit seed extract for its antifungal, antiviral and antibacterial properties. (Do not confuse this with grapeseed extract, a potent antioxidant). Grapefruit seed extract comes in liquid form or capsules. As it has a very sour and bitter taste, it should be mixed into a favorite food or a bit of maple or natural fruit syrup. Grapefruit seed extract has strong action, and only a very few drops are necessary. Consult the directions on the bottle as dose goes by body weight. Capsules are easier to administer as soon as the child is old enough to swallow them.

3. Give nutritional plant enzymes each time the child eats, even snacks. Protease should be the first ingredient listed on the label, along with amylase, lipase and cellulase. Capsules can be opened and the contents mixed with food if the child is too young to swallow capsules. Nutritional plant enzymes can be given indefinitely, but should be continued at least a few weeks past the last symptoms. One or two capsules with meals and one capsule with snacks, depending on body weight is usually sufficient.

4. Eliminate dairy products. This includes all dairy products such as

milk, cheese, yogurt, ice cream, etc. Also eliminate all products containing refined sugar, peanuts and peanut butter. This alone will help the digestive tract improve function because it eliminates the foods that place the greatest demand upon it. If the child has had severe and/or frequent ear infections, assume that any frequently eaten food, such as wheat, corn or eggs can be involved allergically. These foods need only be removed for one month. The milk and sugar products must be restricted for several months and allowed only infrequently after that period of time. Homogenized, pasteurized milk should never be allowed.

5. Use mullein oil ear drops, available at health food stores, nightly for two weeks. Then use the ear drops only if symptoms of ear infection should reappear. A good formula contains mullein oil, hypericum oil and garlic oil.

This program covers only the usual or common case. If your child still demonstrates symptoms after six weeks of adherence to this program, additional advice should be sought. Nearly all children with ear infection will show improvement on this program, but some children have special idiosyncrasies that must be addressed. This program has been successful with hundreds of children with no negative side effects.

Bed-Wetting

Bed-wetting (*nocturnal enuresis*) is a common problem of childhood. Recent statistics show 20% to 25% of children are still affected by bed-wetting at the age of six. This results in tension and anxiety for both the child and the family. The child's self-esteem often suffers. Yet medical reports indicate that there is seldom any physical abnormality with the child. The vast majority of these children have normal urinalysis and normal physical findings, including normal bladder size.

The frequency of bed-wetting tends to decrease as the child grows older with only one or 2% of cases persisting into adulthood. Medical treatment stresses control of the problem rather than treatment. Dr. Robert Schwarz, Associate Professor of Urology, associated with the Department of Pediatrics at Dalhousie University in Halifax,

Nova Scotia, states, "It is not known why some children are bed-wetters." He adds that "laziness" or deliberate bed-wetting is rare and seen only in conjunction with other overt behavioral problems.

There appears to be no correlation between EEG sleep patterns and wetting episodes. Medical management centers on the use of drugs such as tricyclic anti-depressants. Another control method is the electric alarm system, which depends on the child's age and ability to respond to the training measure. However, neither of these methods helps correct underlying biochemical or allergic problems which may be present.

The usual case history is that of an apparently healthy child with no diagnosed physical disturbances of the bladder or urethra, no current urinary infections and no known neurological symptoms. There is often a family history of bed-wetting, on one or both parents' sides. The child toilet trains at a normal age and has no daytime wetting problems. Frequency of bed-wetting ranges from nightly or several times per week to several times per month.

In 1959, an exhaustive study of bed-wetting was conducted which showed that from 83% to 90% of all primary nocturnal enuresis could be controlled by the control of food allergens. In this study, the reactive foods in order of their frequency were milk-60%, wheat-20%, egg-20%, corn-15%, orange-15%, chocolate-15%, and pork, tomato, peanut, seafood, and cinnamon - 5%. James C. Breneman, MD, states, "The most convincing data now shows that food allergies are a major cause of enuresis."

Dr. Breneman was among the first to report that offending foods can cause swelling of the mucosal lining of the bladder, which decreases the internal size or capacity of the bladder. This functional decrease in capacity is only apparent during the times that the offending food is eaten. The overall size of the bladder remains normal, with only the internal volume being decreased. In addition, swelling of the mucosal and muscle layers of the bladder reduces the ability of the bladder to stretch. The internal and external sphincters (valves) of the bladder are also subject to swelling as an allergic response. The usual result is that they are unable to contract tightly and may fatigue more quickly. In the presence of bladder edema, neurologic stimuli is probably more difficult to interpret.

Nichole's Success Story

Nichole, age eight, was having problems with chronic bed-wetting which was still almost a nightly occurrence. This condition was creating a social problem for her as she had reached an age where she wanted to sleep over at her friends' houses, but didn't dare because of the bed-wetting. Her mother had tried everything she could think of to help Nichole. She had taken Nichole to her medical doctor for tests, but had been told that everything was normal.

Testing revealed that Nichole was intolerant to sugar, wheat, beef and mold. She was not digesting her food well. She was also nutrient deficient in vitamins A, C and E and iron. The offending foods were removed from the diet. Nichole was given a nutrient supplement and plant enzymes to take at each meal and an herbal extract to speed up healing of the lining of the intestinal tract. She received chiropractic adjustments directed at improving nerve and body function.

The bed-wetting began to improve by the second week of treatment and had completely ceased by the second month. Nichole showed a lot of motivation to get well, as she had been very embarrassed by the bed-wetting. She followed her diet strictly at first. In Nichole's case sugar appeared to be the trigger that caused the symptoms. She soon found that she could eat almost anything except sugar. On occasion when she drank soda pop, she would have a wet night. Even this disappeared after eight months. Easter came along at this time, and Nichole ate a lot of chocolate Easter eggs. However, this time she did not wet the bed. She found that when she kept consumption of sugar occasional, she no longer wet the bed. She was able to eat all food groups without symptoms. Nichole remained free of bed-wetting.

Although milk is the most common food identified as triggering bed-wetting, it is possible for any food, combination of foods, or food groups to be responsible. Complete elimination of the offending foods is necessary during treatment. Nutritional plant enzymes should be given at each meal and snack, with the dosage depending on the body weight of the child. Yeast overgrowth or local infection of the urethra is also common in many children with bed-wetting problems. A good percentage of these children have a case history of recurrent middle ear infection and have been treated repeatedly with antibiotics. Local genital itchiness, allergies, eczema and ear infections are all symptomatic of yeast infection in children. Lactobacillus acidophilus and bifidus should be given to the child along with abstinence from the offending foods.

Blood sugar imbalance is another commonly associated condition that triggers bed-wetting. However, sugar is not the only problem food. It has been found that any food that reacts allergically can cause changes in blood sugar and lead to bed-wetting.

Help for Bed-wetting
• Eliminate milk and all dairy products
• Eliminate all forms of sugar including honey, maple syrup, desserts
• Eliminate any other food known to trigger an allergic or intolerant reaction
• Supplement with nutritional plant enzymes every time food is eaten
• Culture the colon with probiotics (lactobacillus acidophilus and bifidus)
• Supplement with B-complex containing pantothenic acid and chromium to help stabilize blood sugar levels.

Eczema – The Most Common Skin Problem of Children

Eczema is characterized by itchy, scaly, red, weeping or infected skin. Its typical distribution is on the face, behind the ears, the front of the elbows, back of the knees, wrists and trunk. Sometimes eczema will appear to improve, as the child grows older, only to suddenly reappear.

While medical authorities maintain that the cause of eczema is unknown, they do agree that eczema is the most common skin problem of children and allergic eczema is the most common form.

Medical treatment is directed at controlling the condition, rather than looking for the cause. Zoltan P. Rona, MD, author of *Childhood Illness and the Allergy Connection*, writes, "Dermatologists usually prescribe cortisone-based creams to treat eczema; they rarely consider the systemic cause of a rash, preferring to suppress the symptoms."

Causes or Triggers?

There are many things which may trigger an outbreak of eczema. Sometimes these have been considered, causes, but are really only factors which, when avoided, help to decrease the flare-ups.

Some of these traditional triggers which make eczema worse include:
• excessive scratching of the skin
• moisture, such as sweat
• overheating
• house dust and house mites
• wool or scratchy fabric
• dog or cat dander
• cigarette smoke
• detergent residue in clothes
• soap

While all of the above can exacerbate eczema, they do not cause it. The cause does not start on the skin; the skin is the effect of what is going on internally. The skin is considered the largest organ of the body and it is a major eliminative organ along with the kidneys, bowels, and lungs. Often when the skin erupts in sores, the body is trying to rid itself of internal toxins and metabolic byproducts.

Although eczema is an individualized condition, it nevertheless has common, underlying similarities present in almost all cases. When treatment is directed at this underlying pattern, better results are achieved.

Clinical experience demonstrates that six conditions are nearly always present in children who have eczema.

1. Systemic candidiasis
2. Food allergies and sensitivities
3. Maldigestion
4. Imbalanced colon microflora
5. Poor food choices
6. Nutrient deficiencies

Eczema is multicausal; meaning it has more than one cause. The above conditions are all related, with one thing intertwining with the next, resulting in a pattern of conditions which underlie the eczema. Because of this, it is necessary to do more than one thing to reverse it. While all the causes of eczema may not be known, natural healing offers a more solid solution by working with the underlying conditions that are known.

Eczema Protection Program

While parents of bottle-feeding infants and children with severe eczema should consult professional help before beginning any self-care program, there are some safe, non-toxic measures that can be done at home. Best of all, if other allergic conditions are present, these also tend to improve. Follow the steps of this core program to heal eczema. All steps should be started together and followed for four to five weeks.

1. Eliminate completely from the diet the most common foods associated with eczema. This means not only the foods themselves, but anything that contains these foods. The foods to eliminate are the following: cow's milk and all dairy products, sugar and all sugar products, yeast and all yeast products, wheat, eggs, peanuts and pork. Also eliminate any other food suspected of precipitating a breakout of eczema.

2. Culture the colon with lactobacillus acidophilus and bifidobacteria. Use a good quality powder obtained from your health food store. Probiotic products generally have a pleasant flavor and may be mixed with pure water, a bit of juice, or pureed fruit.

3. Supplement with nutritional plant enzymes which contain at least these four enzymes: protease, amylase, lipase, and cellulase. For children under age two, look for a children's' enzyme formula. Capsules may be opened and mixed with the first bite of food. Enzymes should be taken with each meal and with all snacks. Enzymes break down food particles and help to halt adverse food reactions.

4. Include grapefruit seed extract for its antifungal, antiviral and antibacterial properties. (Do not confuse this with grapeseed extract, a potent antioxidant). Grapefruit seed extract comes in liquid form or capsules. As it has a very sour and bitter taste, it should be mixed into a favorite food or a bit of maple or natural fruit syrup. Grapefruit seed extract has strong action, and only a very few

drops are necessary. Consult the directions on the bottle as dose goes by body weight. Capsules are easier to administer as soon as the child is old enough to swallow them.

5. Supplement with a flaxseed oil blend which contains a balanced mixture of the essential fatty acids, linoleic (Omega 6) and alpha-linolenic (Omega 3). The nutrients of these essential oils are usually deficient in individuals with eczema. Flaxseed oil and evening primrose oil have anti-inflammatory and immune-enhancing effects and studies have shown that over two-thirds of eczema sufferers improve dramatically with the supplementation and topical application of evening primrose oil alone. For best effects, a blend of these important oils is recommended. Children require only one or two teaspoons per day. Eliminate antagonistic oils which include supermarket-processed oils and oils found in margarine, shortenings, salad dressings and packaged foods. Vitamin A and zinc supplementation has also been shown to be very beneficial.

6. Apply calendula cream or gel that contains tea tree oil to the eczematous lesions one to several times a day.

Asthma

Asthma has been increasing in incidence over the last few decades. While no one knows for sure, it is estimated that in the United States, there are nearly 15 million Americans with asthma. Of these, nearly 20% experience limitation of their daily activities. Since 1977, the asthma rate has doubled and asthma has become the most common chronic respiratory disease of children. In Canada, 13% of all students surveyed had current asthma. Canada has concluded that there is a general trend of increased deaths and hospitalizations from asthma recorded in all the industrialized countries of the world. Another startling statistic is that one out of every 12 members of the 1988 U.S. Olympic team was taking medication for asthma.

Medically, asthma is broken down into several types. The most common type of asthma is bronchial asthma, which is caused by a narrowing of the passages that carry air from the throat to the lungs. This narrowing is created by muscle contraction (spasm), local inflammation inducing swelling or the production of excess mucus.

Any or a combination of these three conditions will lead to difficulty breathing and usually wheezing. During a bronchial asthma attack, the bronchi do not allow sufficient air to reach the lungs and the individual begins to labor for breath. Often, the person will feel tightness in the chest and may gasp for air. The face may turn pale, or become gray or blue around the mouth and lips. Many times the person will cough or spit up a considerable amount of mucus. For many people, asthma attacks become chronic.

Asthma is the body's reaction to many kinds of irritants. Therefore, doctors categorize asthma into the following forms:

1. Allergic asthma which is asthma caused by allergens.
2. Non-allergic asthma, often triggered by infection or environmental chemicals.
3. Asthma resulting from emotional or physical situations (such as exercise).
4. Intrinsic asthma which is chronic asthma that is not triggered by allergies and has no obvious cause.

One category missing in the above asthma types and often not recognized by doctors is asthma as a reaction to foods, either allergic or intolerant. Recently, more evidence for this type of trigger is mounting. *The Encyclopedia of Natural Health* lists common problem foods for asthmatics as cow's milk, eggs, peanuts, wheat, citrus fruits and many food additives. James Braly, MD, states, "The provocateur may be a food. Wheat, milk, and eggs are common culprits. In many cases colorings (FD&C Yellow No. 5), preservatives (metasulfites, sodium benzoate), and other chemical additives to food are at fault)."

Ratner and Untracht conducted a study with a group of 500 children with asthma, finding about 5% with clinical reactions to egg white. *Food Allergy and Intolerance* states that "Food allergy is a very important cause of asthma but is often overlooked." It is overlooked because the usual skin (prick) tests are often negative for foods. However, medical studies have found that "immune complexes containing food antigens may be detected in the blood of asthmatic subjects undergoing challenge, and these may trigger bronchoconstriction. The abnormal immune reaction starts in the gut, however..." this is clear evidence that food molecules are capable of triggering off asthma attacks. After citing several more medical studies, the chapter on asthma concludes, "Food intolerance is a very substantial cause of asthma as well as of other symptoms. This fact is very much neglected due to lack of awareness that foods and food additives may be responsible and because skin (prick) tests with foods are often negative or not practicable with food additives. Asthma may be ascribed solely to inhalants or considered to be intrinsic."

Clinical experience has demonstrated that individuals with asthma often have a combination of the following triggers:
• Chronic infection (yeast or fungal, viral, bacterial, or parasitic).
• Food allergy and/or intolerance
• Allergy to inhalants (pollens, grasses, dust, environmental chemicals, etc).

Asthma can be helped to a great extent by the removal of the above stressors. Children especially respond quickly and have a good chance to become well. When beginning any new program, never discontinue any prescribed medication. Any asthma attacks must always be treated promptly with prescribed medication.

The following protocol is best done under the supervision of a licensed health practitioner. The health care provider should have a means of screening an individual for chronic infections including Candida albicans, other fungi such as Aspergillus, viruses, bacteria and parasites and be familiar with natural herbal remedies that help these conditions. Allergic or intolerant foods must also be identified and eliminated from the diet for at least eight weeks. In addition, problem inhalants and chemicals should be avoided as much as possible during treatment.

Clinical experience has shown that most patients suffering from asthma exhibit signs of fungal infection, especially Candida. To a lesser extent, Aspergillus may also be involved in allergic reactions with people who have asthma. Aspergillus can form a fungal ball called an aspergilloma in the lungs or it can appear as an invasive infection which can damage organs of the body such as the lungs, heart, brain, kidney and eyes. Following a good Candida program and diet is usually indicated (see chapter 19). If Aspergillus appears to be involved, add homeopathic Aspergillus to the program. Eliminate all dairy products (except butter) for at least 8 weeks. Also eliminate all forms of sugar and foods containing sugar including honey, molasses, brown sugar, and maple syrup.

In addition, do not include in the diet any other food that appears to be reactive. Nutritional plant enzymes should be included in the program, taken every time the individual eats, including snacks. Nutritional plant enzymes aid in the digestion of food and help to stop allergic reactions. They also help to reduce inflammation, improve circulation, and stimulate the immune system. If several foods appear to be reactive, herbs to help heal the intestinal lining should also be included. These herbs are listed in chapter 19. When the sinuses are involved, natural inhalation therapy with tee tree oil described in Chapter 19 should give relief. Avoid as much as possible breathing in any irritating substances. Chiropractic adjustments are also very helpful and tend to speed up recovery time as well as helping to make breathing easier.

The above program will remove a great deal of stress that the body is experiencing. As asthmatic symptoms begin to improve, individuals usually notice that they require less medication. Many children have been able, over time, to stop their medication altogether. This, however, must always be done under the supervision of your medical doctor.

As conditions within the body improve, this is a good time to add in nutritional supplements to help support the immune system. Use a formula that contains several immune building ingredients such as echinacea, goldenseal, garlic, astragulus, wild indigo, myrrh, boneset, vitamin C with bioflavonoids, vitamin A, beta carotene, B-6, Vitamin E, selenium, zinc, glutathione, coenzyme Q-10, thymus (bovine), spleen (bovine). A good multiple vitamin and mineral supplement is also recommended.

John's Success Story

According to his parents, John, age 5, was "born breathing heavy." He was diagnosed with asthma at the age of 5 months. When John was seen in my office, he was exhibiting a sore throat, infections in both ears, and had a history of diarrhea and colic. He was sensitive to peanuts, chocolate, oats, shellfish, feathers and various pollens. Upon examination, he had the characteristic signs of Candida overgrowth as well as infection with Aspergillus.

John was put on an anti-fungal program which consisted of an anti-fungal supplement, homeopathic Aspergillus, lactobacillus acidophilus and a Candida diet. It was also recommended that he take a vitamin supplement for his throat, ear drops of garlic and mullein oil, and plant enzymes. While on the program, he was asked not to eat the reactive foods of peanuts, chocolate, oats and shellfish. He was also asked not to use a feather pillow.

At his next appointment two weeks later, his parents reported that John was "considerably improved." They expressed amazement at how quickly things had changed after John started the program. The parents stated that John, who had required 2 to 3 puffs of prescription medication per day prior to treatment, had needed only one puff the entire second week! John no longer had throat and ear infection. By the time John finished the 6-week program, he was no longer using the prescription medication. He continued the acidophilus, plant enzymes, and an immune fortifying supplement for another 3 months. Five years later, John has had no reoccurrence of asthma.

Hyperactivity

Many of the same factors that create colic, ear infection and bed-wetting also create hyperactivity, short attention span and behavior and learning problems. In 1950, a typical classroom averaged one hyperactive child. Today there are five or six hyperactive children per classroom. Children with attention deficit hyperactive disorder (ADHD) are disruptive, impulsive, exhibit poor concentration and are easily distracted. They may also be fidgety and irritable and have a variety of learning problems. Studies indicate that 25% to 50% of ADHD children have learning disabilities and around 30% of these children are bed-wetters.

The major areas to address are:
• Poor nutrition and faulty digestion.
• Food allergies and intolerance.
• Environmental toxins.

• Yeast overgrowth and parasites.
• Repeated antibiotics and other medications.

All of the above can adversely affect a child's nervous system re-sulting in various behavioral abnormalities. For example, children with ear infection due to allergic reactions, often become those who are hyperactive, by receiving repeated doses of antibiotics that lead to yeast overgrowth, which in turn produces a leaky gut, allowing aller-gy to emerge and weaken the immune system. This creates toxins which irritate the nervous system. With hyperactivity, elimination of allergens (both food and chemical) in the diet and the addition of plant enzyme therapy is a vital step. The child should also be checked for yeast overgrowth and parasites; and a dietary program should be instituted that is specific for the child.

16

Chemical Allergies

We live in a time of unprecedented environmental change. Because almost everything we eat now contains chemical additives and contaminants, and more toxic and allergic chemicals are added to the air and water, we are stressing to the breaking point our body's ability to dispose of them. Dr. Richard Mackarness writes in his book, *Chemical Allergies*, that, "People at the more susceptible end of the spectrum of adaptability are now cluttering up hospital beds and doctors' surgeries with illnesses which are neither diagnosed correctly nor treated effectively." Dr. Mackarness further states, "It is not logical immediately to prescribe anti-depressant pills for a girl suffering from suicidal depression without first considering whether her depression might be a manifestation of adaptive breakdown to an environmental hazard like instant coffee or cigarettes."

The most important thing to recognize about food additives is that none of them are good for your health. Most additives either cause or have the potential to cause toxic and allergic reactions. The body requires enzymes and nutrients to rid itself of food additives and chemicals. Today, as fewer nutrients are available in foods and the chemical content steadily rises, more people are reacting adversely to these foreign substances. Today we are seeing more and more occurrence of both chemical additives and allergies.

Consider this:

1. Two and a half billion pounds of pesticides are released into the environment each year. Farmers use 60% of these pesticides.
2. Over 4,000 varieties of drugs are fed to animals which produce milk, eggs and meat. About half of all the drugs manufactured in

the United States are given to farm animals, many of them as med-icated feed.

3. Pesticide and drug residues in food are common. Food additives are substances, whether natural or synthetic, which are added to original food substances. Since almost every food in a can, bottle or package contains additives, we can see that over 90% of foods in the supermarket contain additives.

4. Zane R. Gard, MD, reported in the April 1987 issue of the *Townsend Letter*, "Three thousand [chemicals] have been identified as intention-ally added to food supplies and over 700 in drinking water. During food processing and storage more than 10,000 other compounds can become an integral part of many commonly used foods."

5. Each person now consumes 8 to 15 pounds of food additives per year.

6. In the last 45 years. Consumption of chemically altered foods has risen from 10% to 80% of the total diet.

James Braly, MD, writes, "It is now well-established that some of these chemicals actually have the ability to change the digestive process and distort the permeability of the intestinal lining, the last barrier between the outside world and your bloodstream."

Food is the largest single stimulus to the body on a daily basis and, once eaten, the body must process it through a series of enzyme reactions.

Researchers think that it takes several generations to build en-zymes for a new food. Since the ingestion of chemicals and additives is a relatively new phenomenon, it appears certain that we are de-manding that our bodies adapt to such changes at too rapid a pace.

There is little evidence to indicate that sufficient enzymes can be manufactured by the body to metabolize these chemicals. Although the body does has the ability to metabolize (break down) foreign chemicals, how well it performs this function is dependent on two conditions:
• Genetic and inherited ability
• The quantity of chemicals challenging the body

When a foreign chemical enters the body, the body responds in two ways: detoxification and elimination. Detoxification involves chemical processes (oxidation, reduction, and hydrolysis) that begin to render the chemical less toxic to the body. For example, the enzyme alcohol dehydrogenase is necessary to detoxify ethanol. This enzyme requires a molecule of zinc in order to function. A zinc deficient person is unable to effectively process alcohol. The next step is when chemical groups such as glutathione and other sulfur compounds attach to the offending chemical. This serves to increase the size, polarity and solubility of the chemical so that it can be extracted from the body and eliminated in urine, sweat or stool. However, the glutathione and other compounds are lost to the body in this process. The work of detoxification causes the body to use up its nutrients and lose energy in the process. The more the body is overburdened with chemicals to detoxify, the more the nutrient and energy loss. This process has the ultimate effect of increasing nutrient needs. There are three important characteristics of chemical sensitivity:

• Chemical sensitivity can produce any symptom, in any person, at any time. However, the brain is the most common organ involved.

• There is a vast range of individual susceptibility. For example, a family exposed to a certain chemical may have one member with headaches, another with joint pains, a third member with flu-like symptoms and still others with no symptoms at all.

• Chemical sensitivity may produce a spreading effect, whereby exposure to one chemical will produce susceptibility to other chemicals.

When substances cannot be metabolized efficiently, they place stress on the body in the form of toxicity, leading to negative reactions. Some of the toxic effects of additives are known; and the consumer, whether suffering from allergies or any other health problem should be aware of these negative effects.

Four substances found in foods are especially prevalent and pertinent to people with allergy.

The Big Four: Sulfites, Tartrazine, BHA / BHT and MSG

1. Sulfites

Sulfites come in many forms — sodium bisulfate and sodium or potassium metabisulfite, sulfur dioxide, sodium sulfite, potassium sulfite and bisulfate. Sulfites are used as preservatives and antioxidants. They keep fresh food from turning brown. Because allergy sufferers and asthmatics are particularly sensitive to them and because they have led to seventeen confirmed deaths in the United States, some laws have been passed limiting their use. However, sulfites are still allowed in many products. The most common products are wine, beer, fresh vegetables and fruit, citrus drinks, potato products such as chips and fries, fish and shrimp, dried fruits, fruit snacks and many frozen items such as potato products and TV dinners.

Mild to moderate symptoms from sulfites include hives, weakness, difficulty breathing, dizziness, abdominal pain, diarrhea and vomiting. Severe reactions can result in anaphylaxis and death. Sulfites have caused tumors in rats.

Hundreds of medications contain sulfites. It is ironic that while asthmatics are particularly sensitive to sulfites, many bronchodilators contain up to 6ppm (parts per million) of sulfur dioxide. When inhaled, this is enough to cause bronchospasm. Other drugs that contain sulfites include heart medications, steroids, antibiotics, pain medicines and muscle relaxants.

The average daily intake of sulfites with food eaten at home is 2 to 3 mg per day. In contrast, the average restaurant meal contains an estimated 25 to 200 mg of sulfites. In addition to their allergenic potential, sulfites destroy vitamin B1 in foods.

2. Tartrazine or Yellow Dye #5

Most food dyes are known carcinogens. They are also potential allergens. Tartrazine imparts a yellow color to food. It is a synthetic dye derived from coal tar. Several tons of food dyes are consumed every year. The chemical structure of Yellow Dye #5 is nearly identical to that of aspirin. People who are allergic to aspirin may also be allergic to this dye.

Soft drinks, candy and desserts are particularly high in tartrazine. About 500 drugs contain this dye as a coloring agent. The estimated average intake is 15 mg per day. However, some individuals or children consuming excess soft drinks and candy have intakes up to 150 mg per day. Tartrazine is a causative agent in bronchial asthma.

Other common foods which contain this dye are as following: cheese, cake mixes, frostings, canned vegetables, chewing gum, fruit juices, macaroni and cheese, meat tenderizer, puddings, salad dressings, ice cream, ice milk, sherbet, milk, jams and jellies with pectin, ketchup, pickles, relishes, canned fruit, butter, margarine, baked goods, Popsicles™, fruit drinks, gelatins, colored cereals, banana and lime flavoring, mustards, smoked fish, salted anchovy, salted shrimp, wine coolers and liqueurs. Although tartrazine may be used in Canada and the United States, it has been banned for use in Austria, Finland, Sweden, and Norway.

3. BHA and BHT

These preservatives and antioxidants were designed for use in petroleum products and rubber, but found their way into breakfast cereals. BHA and BHT can affect the nervous system and are known to cause behavioral problems in children. At levels now permitted in foods, there is evidence that BHT may convert hormones and oral contraceptives into carcinogenic agents. BHT has been banned from all foods in England.

People with urticaria (hives) and asthma often react allergically to BHA and BHT. Testing in rats demonstrated that BHA and BHT inhibited growth, caused weight loss and damaged the liver, kidneys and testicles, caused blindness and elevated blood cholesterol levels. In humans, BHT accumulates in fat tissue.

Common foods that contain these chemicals are cereals, instant potato flakes, frozen dinners, baked goods, fruit drinks, fats, oils, lard, margarine, chewing gum, citrus oil flavors and many others.

4. MSG: Monosodium glutamate

MSG has an interesting history. Its usefulness as a flavor enhancer of foods is unequaled by any other additive. On the other hand, it is associated with a long list of negative health effects. In 1978 MSG was removed from baby food because it was shown to cause damage to the brain stem in infants. MSG masquerades under the names of hydrolyzed vegetable protein, autolyzed yeast, hydrolyzed yeast, vegetable powder, or natural flavors.

MSG occurs in larger amounts in foods than other additives, often in gram amounts rather than milligrams. The average daily intake is one gram. A typical Chinese meal contains five to ten grams of MSG. Although MSG is ordinarily associated with Chinese food, nearly all restaurants use MSG.

Over 20 million people in the United States are highly sensitive to MSG. If the dose is high enough, everyone will react to MSG.

Children are very sensitive to MSG. Exposure over time can result in behavioral disorders or impaired intellect. Brain damage is possible with prolonged exposure to high enough dosages.

Common symptoms of MSG usage include headache, asthma and chest pains. Other symptoms include: diarrhea, blurred vision, fatigue, hot flashes, numbness around the face, sweating, palpitations and urinary discomfort.

Fast food restaurants are particularly heavy users of MSG. Practically everything that is breaded contains MSG. This includes fried chicken and chicken nuggets, fried fish, cheese balls and sticks, fried zucchini, onion rings and breaded meats such as pork chops and veal Parmesan. The product Accent™ is pure MSG. Who would suspect that MSG might be added to some brands of water-packed tuna or dry roasted nuts? Soy sauce, bouillon and canned and dry soups are more obvious sources. Other foods commonly containing MSG are ketchup, frozen dinners, frozen vegetables, canned and cured meats and noodle dishes.

Vitamin B6 is necessary for the metabolism of MSG. Therefore, MSG has the effect of causing vitamin B6 deficiency. B6 in sufficient quantities has been known to stop reactions to MSG.

Other Additives: Alcohol, Alginates, Artificial Flavors, Aspartame, Benzoic Acid/Sodium Benzoate, Nitrates/Nitrites and Propyl Gallate

Alcohol

Alcohol contributes to food allergy in several ways:

It increases intestinal permeability, thereby allowing potential allergenic substances to be absorbed into the blood stream and precipitate reactions. It is a major contributor to the leaky gut syndrome.

Alcohol is very rapidly absorbed from the stomach and intestine. This rapid absorption coupled with the fact that alcohol carries with it the reactivity of the food from which it was made, makes it a potent allergen. This is what makes it a powerful addictant, which we commonly observe as alcoholism. For example, in clinical studies, social drinkers who become inebriated on as little as two drinks of beer or whisky were found to be sensitive to corn, wheat, malt, barley, rye or yeast. Most alcoholic beverages are not required to carry on their labels a list of the ingredients, making it difficult for the consumer to know what they contain, or from what they were made.

Corn, barley, rye, wheat, oats and rice are the common grains used in the production of straight and blended whisky and vodka. The first three are generally used to make gin. Corn and barley are the usual grains used in beer and ale. Other ingredients in alcoholic beverages such as cane sugar, malt or yeast can also produce allergic reactions. If a person is allergic to the grain from which the alcohol was made, the reaction can be exaggerated or more extreme than a reaction to the grain itself due to the rapid absorption of the alcohol.

Some people react to the pesticide residues contained in the beverage. Pesticides, such as the chlorinated hydrocarbons, which came into use after 1945, can cause symptoms such as redness in the face, hyperactivity, headache and depression. In addition to the fact that alcohol is absorbed rapidly, it tends to cause more rapid absorption of some foods.

When alcoholics stop drinking, they tend to substitute the edible form of their specific addictants. Most alcoholics are allergic to corn. When they stop drinking, they substitute corn sugar found in candy, cookies and doughnuts or other products containing corn sugar, dextrose or glucose. This continues both the addiction and the craving.

Alginates

Many forms of alginate are used in processed foods. There is ammonium, calcium, potassium, sodium and glycol alginate, and there are also algin derivatives. Alginates stabilize and impart a creamy texture to foods and are found in infant formula, ice cream, salad dressings, cheese spreads, cream cheese, calorie-reduced margarine, and frozen dinners. Alginates have been shown to inhibit the absorption of essential nutrients in test animals. Alginates are also being tested in relation to reproductive problems.

Artificial Flavors

Approximately 2000 chemicals are used in a variety of combinations to produce specific flavors. Common flavors are butyl acetate, benzaldehyde, methyl salicylates and benzyl alcohol. Flavors, even those termed natural have been known to cause allergies and hyperactivity in children, although depression, migraine headaches and reproductive problems have also been associated with them. Symptoms from artificial flavors can be widespread in the body. Skin disorders, respiratory problems, blood abnormalities, gastrointestinal upsets and neurological disturbances have all been reported.

Aspartame

More lawsuits have been launched against aspartame in the length of time it has been on the market than any other artificial sweetener. It was first approved for use in 1981. 1985 used more than 800 million pounds used each year in the United States. Aspartame is the technical name for the brand names, NutraSweet™, Equal™, Spoonful™, and Equal-Measure™. Aspartame accounts for over 75% of the adverse reactions to food additives reported to the U.S. Food and Drug Administration (FDA).

Many of these symptoms, including seizures and death, were reported in a February 1994, Department of Health and Human Services report. 90 different symptoms were documented in the report as being caused by aspartame. Symptoms include headaches, migraines, dizziness, nausea, muscle spasms, weight gain, rashes, depression, fatigue, irritability, tachycardia, insomnia, vision problems, hearing loss, heart palpitations, breathing difficulties, anxiety attacks, slurred speech, loss of taste, tinnitus, vertigo, memory loss, and joint pain. Recognized allergic symptoms are severe itching, hives and swelling of the lips, mouth, tongue and throat. Studies show that a high intake of aspartame could cause brain damage in infants. For this reason, some obstetricians advise mothers not to consume products with aspartame during pregnancy or breast-feeding. In addition, some chronic conditions are thought to be triggered or made worse by aspartame. These conditions include brain tumors, multiple sclerosis, epilepsy, chronic fatigue syndrome, Parkinson's disease,

Alzheimer's disease, mental retardation, lymphoma, birth defects, fibromyalgia and diabetes.

Aspartame is made up of three chemicals: aspartic acid, phenylalanine, and methanol.

Aspartic acid (40% of aspartame)

When ingested in its free form (unbound to proteins) it significantly raises the blood plasma level of aspartate and glutamate. Too much aspartate or glutamate can kill neurons by allowing too much calcium to enter the cells. This influx triggers excessive amounts of free radicals, which kill the cells. It has been found that excess aspartate and glutamate can cross the blood brain barrier (which normally protects the brain from toxins). Neurons are destroyed as aspartate and glutamate seep into the brain. Up to 75% of neural cells in an area of the brain can be killed before any clinical symptoms appear.

Phenylalanine (50% of aspartame)

Ingesting aspartame, especially along with carbohydrates can lead to excess levels of phenylalanine in the brain. Excessive levels of phenylalanine in the brain can cause the levels of serotonin (a neurotransmitter) in the brain to decrease, leading to emotional disorders such as depression.

Methanol (wood alcohol) (10% of aspartame)

The absorption of methanol into the body is sped up when free methanol is ingested. Free methanol is created from aspartame when it is heated to above 86° F or 30° C. Examples are soft drinks containing aspartame, which are not refrigerated in warm climates or when a food product such as a gelatin dessert is made with boiling water.

Methane toxicity mimics multiple sclerosis and because of this, some people have been diagnosed in error as having multiple sclerosis. Symptoms of methanol poisoning include: headaches, ear buzzing, dizziness, nausea, gastrointestinal disturbances, weakness, vertigo, chills, memory lapses, numbness and shooting pains in the extremities, behavioral problems, and neuritis. Vision problems are common and include misty vision, blurring of vision, retinal damage and blindness.

An EPA assessment of methanol states that it "is considered a cumulative poison due to the low rate of excretion once it is absorbed. In the body, methanol is oxidized to formaldehyde and formic acid; both of these metabolites are toxic." The recommended limit is 7.9 mg/day. A one-liter beverage sweetened with aspartame may contain about 56 mg. of methanol.

Foods That Commonly Contain Aspartame

Breath mints	Pharmaceuticals and supplements
Cereals	Soft drinks
Cocoa mixes	Sugar-free chewing gum
Coffee beverages	Sugar-free labeled foods
Frozen desserts	Tabletop sweeteners
Gelatins	Tea beverages
Juice beverages	Topping mixes
Milk drinks	Wine coolers
Multiple vitamins (some brands of children's chewable)	Yogurt

Benzoic Acid and Sodium Benzoate

These additives are used as preservatives and anti-fungal agents. They affect the nervous system and are involved in allergic reactions such as asthma, skin rashes, red eyes, stomach irritations and hyperactivity in children. Benzoic acid has been shown to impair the absorption of nutrients. Benzoic acid is used in fruit juices, jams, jellies, mincemeat, pickles, relishes, catsup, and tomato paste.

Nitrates and Nitrites

These are used primarily as preservatives in cured meats to which they impart a pink color. Nitrites react with secondary amines found in foods containing protein to form nitrosamines. Very small amounts of some nitrosamines can cause cancer in animals. Dr. William Lijinsky, an internationally recognized authority on nitrites and cancer, considers nitrites in meat to be the most dangerous food additives today and they are major contributors to cancer. He feels that the nitrate and nitrite used in luncheon meats, ham, sausages, bacon, wieners and bologna pose a significant risk to children.

Propyl Gallate

This additive is known to precipitate allergic and asthmatic reactions. It is found in frozen dinners, gravy mixes, turkey sausage, lard, shortening, dehydrated potato products, chewing gum, margarine, citrus oils, and breakfast cereals. It is used as an antioxidant to keep fats from becoming rancid. Studies completed in 1981 by the National Cancer Institute found numerous suggestions of cancer in mice and rats.

Common Drugs

These may weaken the intestinal membranes and make them more permeable, leading to increased susceptibility to allergy. Heavy or prolonged drug usage can damage the intestines. Here is a list of common drugs, of concern.

Aspirin	Fiorinal
Bufferin	Heparin
Butazoladin	Indocin
Clinoril	Motrin or Ibuprofen
Cortisone	Naprosyn
Coumadin	Prednisone
Dolobid	Tanderil
Excedrin	Tolectin
Fenoprin	

Why Drug Therapy will Never Solve Chemical Sensitivity

Chemical sensitivity occurs primarily by an overload of chemicals in the tissues that the body had been unable to eliminate. Drugs are also chemicals and an individual with a compromised system is often made worse by additional drug use. New symptoms may emerge because the overloaded system is further stressed.

It is almost prophetic that what was evident fifty years ago, still holds true today. In 1951, Dr. G. Roche Lynch, pathologist and toxicologist and a world authority on forensic medicine opened a conference on *Problems Arising from the Use of Chemicals in Food* with the statement

215

When one peruses the formidable list of substances embraced by this conference, one is struck by the fact that, however necessary these substances are today, not one of them is of the slightest value to the nutrition of the human organism...we know so little about many food additives, and what we do know tends to raise one's doubts rather than allay them.

17

How Thoughts and Emotions Affect Allergy

How do thoughts influence the body? While not all the mechanisms are known, some of the influencing pathways have been discovered. Documentation on how thoughts control internal body functions is accumulating.

Scientist Cleve Backster pioneered research on the idea that there is electrical activity at the cellular level and that this electrical activity can be influenced by thoughts. Using human cells that he had scraped from the roof of the mouth, Backster perfected a method of electrically charging them so they could be monitored with electroencephalogram-type instruments measuring their net electrical potential. Backster then demonstrated that these cells were capable of reacting when the donor was emotionally stressed.

In one case, a female donor of mouth cells reacted emotionally when she watched circumstances leading to a rape scene on television. Even though her mouth cells were being monitored half a mile away, the cells reacted with sharp swings on the recording graph at the exact time of the rape scene. In another example, a male donor was asked to watch a war scene while his mouth cells were being monitored. As he emotionally reacted to the scene of a plane crash, his mouth cells recorded a change on the recording graph.

If emotionally charged thoughts are capable of changing electrical impulses of cells, which are, located half a mile away from the body, thoughts are certainly capable of influencing cells still located in the body.

Thoughts can be generated by external or internal stimuli and thought generation is believed to occur when electrons change orbit. The body is made up of atoms. Atoms contain both electrons and protons with negative and positive charges. The electrons revolve within the atom in spatial domains known as orbitals. Each orbital possesses a specific frequency and energetic characteristics. When energy of a specific frequency (a stimulus) is delivered to the electron, it will excite or boost it into the next highest orbital. When this occurs with enough electrons, a thought may be created or intensified.

Once generated, where do the thoughts go? Guyton's *Textbook of Medical Physiology* tells us that, "When a person experiences some powerful depressing or exciting thought, a portion of the signal is transmitted into the hypothalamus."

The hypothalamus is comprised of neurological tissue lying at the lower portion of the brain. It is so small it composes less than 1% of the total brain mass, yet it is responsible for an immense number of vital body functions. The hypothalamus influences the heart rate, arterial blood pressure, body temperature, thirst, hunger and satiety, uterine contractions and water excretion. It also controls the pituitary gland, known as the master gland of the body, releasing hormones into the blood stream in response to stimuli. Thoughts can be translated into numerous neurological and hormonal stimuli, which can reach any part of the body. In the past, most of these functions have been considered to be "autonomic" or taking place without conscious control.

The hypothalamus, once thought to be a gland, is actually a tiny extension of the brain, which has one very unique characteristic. It is the only part of the brain that has direct blood contact. The rest of the brain and the bones of the skull have protective membranes called the blood-brain barrier. A series of transport mechanisms in this membrane protect the brain from small variations in the composition of the blood. For example, large protein particles cannot enter the brain but proteins in the form of amino acids can.

The transport mechanisms select what can enter the brain and what cannot. Alcohol and steroid hormones readily penetrate the blood-brain barrier.

The hypothalamus, however, deals directly with the blood and all its constituents. It acts like a thermostat taking information from the blood and secreting hormones in response. Besides thought stimulation, the constituents of the blood are a major stimulant to the hypothalamus. What substances are in the blood depends largely on what you choose to eat and how well you digest and absorb it. It is not specifically known what adverse effects undigested particles of food, residues of drugs or chemicals, or inflammatory products of allergic reactions, such as histamine, have on the hypothalamus. However, it seems apparent that if abnormal particles reach this area through the blood, an alarm response of the hypothalamus may send abnormal signals to the rest of the body. This altered information may in turn compromise normal body functions.

Guyton states in the *Textbook of Medical Physiology*,

> Even the concentrations of nutrients, electrolytes, water and various hormones in the blood excite or inhibit various portions of the hypothalamus. Thus, the hypothalamus is a collecting center for information conveyed with the internal well-being of the body.

Where does this information sent by the hypothalamus go? Most of it goes straight to the pituitary gland. Nearly all of the pituitary secretions are controlled either by hormone stimulation or nerve stimulation from the hypothalamus. Hormones arriving through blood vessels control the anterior pituitary, and the posterior pituitary is controlled by nerve fibers from the hypothalamus. Nerve signals reach the hypothalamus from nearly all-possible sources in the nervous system. With a direct blood vessel connection and a direct nerve connection to the pituitary, the entire body is thus influenced. With portions of thought signals being directed through the hypothalamus, we have a real physical body-mind connection.

The internal functions in the body occur, for the most part, without your conscious thought. However, you do have control over the basic mechanism by what you give the hypothalamus to evaluate. Stimuli reach the hypothalamus as an end result of what you think, eat, and drink.

Dr. Candice Pert finds another pathway that provides answers to the question of how our thoughts and emotions affect our health in a fascinating new book, *Molecules of Emotion*. Dr. Pert has pioneered research on how the chemicals inside our bodies form a dynamic information network, which links the body and mind and establish the biomolecular basis for our emotions. Candice Pert, PhD, is a Research Professor in the Department of Physiology and Biophysics at Georgetown University Medical Center in Washington, D.C.

According to Dr. Pert, every cell of the body has millions of receptors floating around on its surface. Messenger molecules called neuropeptides (strings of amino acids, the building blocks of protein) link to these very specific receptor sites, conveying information. These strings of amino acids are capable of forming an infinite number of neuropeptides and it now appears that these messenger molecules can run everything in the body. Peptide molecules are being released from one place and diffusing all over the body and are stimulating the receptors that are on the surface of distant cells.

While neuropeptides originally were believed to reside in a specific area of the body, such as the brain, scientists during the 1980s discovered that nearly all of them are found in all areas of the body and that their primary role is to mediate intercellular communication throughout the body. Cells are constantly signaling other cells through the release of neuropeptides which then bind with receptor sites on other cells. The signaled cells respond by making changes, which are then fed back to the peptide-secreting cell as information. This tells the original cell how much more of the peptide to produce. This very rapid feedback loop is how cells communicate information throughout the body.

Although historically emotions have been considered as psychological, Dr. Pert now feels that these peptides and their receptors are the material manifestation of emotions because emotions appear to mobilize them. When neuropeptides are received at the receptor site, there is a physical attachment process between the peptide and the receptor. As this binding process occurs, a cascade of reactions begins to happen. Ions start pouring in, many changes happen, and the brain receptors perceive what is happening as emotions.

The receptors on the cells are dynamic, wiggling, vibrating energy molecules that are changing their shape from millisecond to millisecond, and also changing what they are attached to. One moment they may be attached to one protein in the membrane and the next moment they can be attached to another. In this dynamic, fluid system, the chemicals that mediate emotion and the receptors for those chemicals are found in almost every cell in the body. Moods and attitudes transform themselves into the physical realm through the emotions, which affect the organs and tissues of the body.

Immune System Link

Recent discoveries reveal that the surface of lymphocytes and monocytes, primary cells involved in immune function, are covered with receptors for neuropeptides. This comprises a tangible immune system link.

Although feelings and thoughts may seem to be intangible, the brain is active anytime that we are thinking or feeling anything. That activity can then lead to a number of changes in the body, which demonstrate that the brain and immune system are communicating with each other all the time. One study at UCLA used actors and actresses who were told to think about a scenario and then generate in their own minds the feeling that comes with it. While they did this, their hormones in the blood were tested and changes could be seen in some hormones in addition to subtle changes in the immune system, depending on what they were feeling. Through the receptors located on immune cells, emotional fluctuations and emotional status can directly influence the probability that a person will get sick or be well.

Dr. Pert explains this concept... "Like information, then, the emotions travel between the two realms of mind and body, as the peptides and their receptors in the physical realm, and as the feelings we experience and call emotions in the nonmaterial realm." Doctors estimate that each person generates 70 thousand thoughts a day.

Dr. M.T. Morter, Jr., author of *The Healing Field*, states that thoughts are energy. He explains, "By understanding that mental activity generates energy and that this energy is transformed into the energy fields of the body, we can understand why thoughts and the mind are so important in gaining, restoring, or maintaining physical health."

18

Energy Allergy: Introducing Electromagnetic Hypersensitivity

Probably the most fascinating and controversial subject relating to health today is the emergence of energy medicine and the recognition of energy illnesses.

Many doctors regard energy medicine as incompatible with existing medical opinion. Robert O. Becker, MD, explains the differing philosophies in his book Cross Currents.

The proponents of orthodox medicine...the kind taught in medical schools and promoted by the Medical Association (AMA) and the Food and Drug Administration (FDA)...are absolutely convinced that the body is simply a machine that cannot heal itself, and the only appropriate therapies are powerful drugs and mechanical technologies. Proponents of energy medicine, on the other hand, believe that the body is more than a machine, and that it is capable not only of healing itself but also of performing other actions that lie completely outside the realm of established science. The latter practitioners believe that an appropriate therapy is one that either encourages the body's own energetic systems or that adds external energy to those systems.

Alongside this divergence of opinion within the medical establishment, doctors in many parts of the world have gone ahead with measuring electrical currents and studying the electrical fields of the body. Much of this work has been done in Russia and to a lesser extent elsewhere in Europe. Because of recently developed instruments, Western scientists are becoming more involved in research of this type. Through this research, it has been discovered that the body has both electrical and magnetic properties.

You are probably familiar with modern diagnostic machines that measure electrical impulses. The electrocardiogram measures electrical impulses of the heart and the electroencephalogram measures electrical waves and activity of the brain. The brain shows continuous electrical activity. Brain waves, as recorded at the surface of the head, vary in intensity from zero to 300 millivolts. Their frequency range is from one cycle every several seconds to 50 or more cycles per second.

In his book Blueprint for Immortality, Harold Saxton Burr writes, "There are electrical properties wherever there is life."

Guyton's *Textbook of Medical Physiology* states:

Electrical potentials exist across the membranes of all cells of the body and some cells, such as nerve cells and muscle cells, are excitable, that is, capable of self-generation of electrochemical impulses at their membranes and in some instances, employment of these impulses to transmit signals along the membranes.

The body is made up of atoms with positive and negative charges in motion. Physics tells us that any time there is a flow of electrons, a magnetic field will be produced in the space around it. Using this law, the motion of ions (atoms with a positive or negative charge) inside the body would generate weak magnetic fields. This can be illustrated by the flow of electric currents in the brain, which produces a magnetic field around the head.

The development of the super-conducting quantum interference device (SQUID) around 1970 led to the discovery of this magnetic field in the space around the human head. The SQUID can measure the magnetic field from several feet away from the head! More recently, scientists have also been able to record the magnetic field associated with the nerve impulse itself.

It has been known that nerves transmit information throughout the body by electrical and chemical means. Hormones (chemical messengers) carry messages from one gland to another and to other parts of the body. Electromagnetic waves, which move with the speed of light, are dependent upon the presence of minerals, protons, and electrons.

Now we are beginning to see that electromagnetic waves carry information capable of communicating between organs, tissues and cells. Dr. Becker backs up this idea. He writes, "Magnetic and electromagnetic fields have energy, can carry information, and are produced by electrical current."

Anything that influences the cell over time will ultimately influence the rest of the body because cells make up the tissues that make up the glands and organs. Cells are fantastically complex. In a human, a single living cell performs over 50,000 different biochemical reactions. Its DNA molecule carries billions of bits of data and contains around 100,000 genes of which 500 are actively producing around 500 different proteins. These numerous biochemical reactions support and maintain the basic life system of the body.

According to Dr. F.A. Popp, a German physician, the amount of information being transmitted per second by just one cell of the body is so great that it would take a hundred years to read it if it were printed. Dr. Popp has shown that "transmitters and receivers" exist in the double helix of the DNA of the cell nucleus. The natural vibrational frequencies of the body are controlled by the positive and negative magnetic fields.

If there is an imbalance in electromagnetic radiation in an organ or tissue, function of that organ or tissue is disturbed. Many scientists now believe that disease, including allergy, can first be detected as a disturbance of the normal flow and balance of energy in the body. If this disturbance continues long enough, changes eventually manifest themselves in the physical tissues.

It appears that just as wrong food can lead to disease, so can wrong electromagnetic waves. Researchers have found that each organ in the body has its own electromagnetic wave frequency. If for any reason the electromagnetic waves are disturbed and the body is unable to correct the disturbance, the frequency of the waves is changed. If it remains changed for a long enough time, pathology develops in the tissues. In other words, abnormal waves develop when the normal waves are blocked or impeded.

The early symptoms of allergy often begin as small shifts in the pattern of the body's energy.

Dr. Kenyon, in Liverpool, England, has studied this phenomenon for a number of years. He believes that the body can detect a harmful substance within its field and will react by producing minute changes in its electrical responses. Also, if an organ in the body is unhealthy, it is unable to maintain a normal supply of energy and its deficiency can be measured. According to Dr. Kenyon, allergy is primarily an electrical phenomenon, and if it continues long enough, it will eventually produce changes in the blood and other tissues.

Since every cell in the body produces energy and has a polarity, energy is the fundamental principle that underlies everything that happens in the body, including biochemical changes. The flow of energy in the body regulates and controls all body processes including the utilization of nutritional substances and the function of the immune system.

Research in biomagnetics has established that a proper balance between the positive and negative magnetic poles in the human body is necessary for health and life itself. Each cell in the body is itself a weak magnet with a positive and negative pole. If a balance is to be maintained between these poles, then we must ask the question, how do these electromagnetic poles become disturbed in humans?

It appears that some of the more common stressors are toxins and chemicals in the food and environment. These, along with allergens, nutritional deficiencies, bacterial and viral infections, all carry a positive magnetic charge that when prolonged can unbalance the positive and negative relationship necessary for health. These stressors may lead to magnetic energy imbalance, which results in physical and emotional illnesses. Although less recognized, the amount of environmental radiation that the body is exposed to on a daily basis has become an increasingly common stressor. This environmental radiation is termed electropollution or electromagnetic contamination.

The natural pulsing frequency of the earth has been determined to be about 7.9 cycles per second. This is also the healthy vibrational frequency of the human body as a whole. Individual organs have their individual frequencies. For instance, the frequency of the brain at rest has been determined to be 1 to 2 cycles per second; awake is 8 to 12 cycles per second; and during concentration is 18 to 22 cycles per second. It is thought that the normal electromagnetic fields of the body are disturbed when the body is exposed over time to other frequencies.

Man-made radiation produces frequencies that are not found in nature, and which are not present in the normal electromagnetic spectrum of the earth. We are all aware that X-rays are damaging to human cells. X-rays are high frequency, ionizing radiation that can cause cancer and genetic changes. However, we are not so familiar with other forms of man-made radiation. We can't see, hear, taste or smell radiation, and consequently tend not to be aware of it.

According to Dr. Robert O. Becker, we are now existing in a "world of energy," the majority of which is man-made radiation which has never before existed on the earth. Every person is bathed every hour of the day and night in a continuous flood of electromagnetic fields with a broad range of frequencies. The density of radio waves around us is now 100 million to 200 million times the natural level reaching us from the sun.

Dr. Becker describes the new electromagnetic environment in which we live.

In addition, new technologies have appeared. Commercial telephone and television satellite transmitters and relays blanket the Earth from 25,000 miles out in space. Military satellites cruise by every point on Earth once an hour, and from their altitude of only 250 miles, they bounce radar beams off its surface to produce images for later 'downloading' over their home countries. New TV and FM stations come on the air weekly. The industry has placed in the hands of the public such gadgets as citizen-band radios and cellular telephones.

Engineers propose gigantic solar-power stations in space, which would relay the electrical energy to Earth by means of enormously powerful microwave beams. Electrical power transmission lines are operating at millions of volts and thousands of amperes of current. Military services of every country use all parts of the electromagnetic spectrum for communications and surveillance, and the use of electromagnetic energy as an antipersonnel weapon is being studied.

Dr. Becker further states:

The scientific evidence leads to only one conclusion: that exposure of living organisms to abnormal electromagnetic fields results in significant abnormalities in physiology and function."

As little as 100 years ago, humans were exposed to only the earth's magnetic field. Less than four generations later, there is bombardment of man-made radiation. So much so, that Dr. Becker feels "We have almost reached a state by which the entire electromagnetic spectrum has been filled up with man-made frequencies." One thing is for sure; no human being has yet lived their entire life surrounded by computers and cellular telephones.

What is Electromagnetic Hypersensitivity?

Electromagnetic hypersensitivity is an environmentally triggered illness, which produces neurological, and allergic-type symptoms brought on by exposure to electromagnetic fields from the environment. There can be a wide range in the degree of sensitivity exhibited by afflicted individuals and many are primarily sensitive to just certain frequencies of electromagnetic radiation. Electromagnetic hypersensitivity is becoming a serious public health concern and the incidence is growing. Awareness is increasing that humans are responding to electromagnetic radiation in a variety of ways.

What are the Common Sources of Electromagnetic Radiation?

Electromagnetic fields are invisible fields of energy produced whenever electric current is flowing. Here is a list of common sources.

Computer monitors

Automobiles with computerized equipment
Cellular telephones
Clock radios
Copying and fax machines
Dimmer switches
Electric blankets
Electric calculators
Electric heaters
Electrical distribution panels and ventilation fans
Electronic security systems
Electric stoves
Fluorescent lights
Freezers
Halogen lamps
High voltage power lines
Household electrical appliances
Indoor and outdoor electrical supply cables (underground and overhead)
Low energy lamps
Microwave ovens
Refrigerators
Telephone answering machines
Television
Vacuum cleaners
Waterbed heaters

Is There Proof?

Many authorities maintain, despite the research, that there is no definite proof to link ill health with exposure to electromagnetic radiation. They feel that a precisely defined explanation of how electromagnetic fields cause ill health is needed and that this link must be further substantiated by studies from more researchers. However, it is already scientifically apparent that there is some kind of connection between electrical equipment and health problems.

In 1964, a Russian researcher conducting experiments on rabbits reported cell death in areas of the brain in rabbits exposed to electromagnetic radiation. Many studies on professions with high exposure to electromagnetic fields have been published. A Swedish study reported an 80% higher cancer risk for employees in electrically exposed occupations such as electricians, technical engineers, kitchen personnel and machine and motor mechanics. Laboratory tests have shown that magnetic fields at certain frequencies encourage cancer cells to divide.

In 1992, the US government authorized a 5-year, $65 million program on electromagnetic field research and public information. New York and California have also sponsored research on electromagnetic fields. In 1997, the American Academy of Environmental Medicine co-sponsored an International symposium titled Bioelectricity with electromagnetic hypersensitivity included as one of the topics presented. The Swedish Association for the ElectroSensitive (FEB), founded in 1987, is among the largest in the world. Its active support group, consisting of around 2000 members, targets support for the electrically injured and helps to create understanding for their problems.

Dr. William Rae, founder of the Environmental Health Center in Dallas, Texas has tested patients with neurological and allergic symptoms by exposing them to a spectrum of electromagnetic fields without the patients' conscious awareness. Dr. Rae has found a consistent sensitivity to specific frequencies in most patients he has tested.

Other evidence that man-made radiation affects human physiology and function is seen in the following examples. Microwave radiation exposure has been linked to cataract formation. Parts of the body especially vulnerable to microwave radiation are the eye, gall-

229

bladder, digestive tract and testes. Dr. Becker states that all microwave ovens emit an average of 120 microwatts near the door.

Reports of the hazard of living near high tension power lines have been creeping in for the last thirty years. One of the most famous studies ever done on the relationship of childhood leukemia and the effects of the high tension power lines appeared in The New Yorker magazine in June 1989. The study cited a two-to-three-fold increase in leukemia rates for children who lived in homes near high current lines.

Still more adverse biological effects have been reported. Dr. John Ott discovered that red blood cells clump together when in close proximity to a visual display terminal. Visual display terminals have also been linked to conditions such as altered cell growth, altered metabolism of protein, carbohydrates and fats, increased cancers and leukemia and miscarriages.

A New York study in 1987 demonstrated that exposure to power lines and radiation from household appliances can increase the rate at which cancer cells grow and can produce long-lasting behavior alterations and changes in brain neurotransmitters.

Dr. Daniel B. Lyle of Loma Linda, California, reported that exposure of human T-cell lymphocytes (the immune system's killer cells) to a 60 Hz electric field for 48 hours significantly reduced their ability to fight foreign invaders. This is evidence of a direct link between common electrical fields and the immune system.

There is also evidence that low frequency fields interfere with the rate at which cells release and absorb calcium. Dr. Ross Adey concludes that low frequency electromagnetic fields can jam the communication signals between cells.

While the debate on exactly how electromagnetic fields affect living tissue will undoubtedly go on for years as further research is conducted, thousands of people from around the world are reporting adverse.

Length of exposure is a critical factor: the longer the exposure, the more the potential to cause harm. Appliances such as hand-held electric hair dryers and electric shavers provide short exposure, compared to constant exposure to high voltage power lines located near a home.

Many persons experience an abrupt onset of symptoms when exposed to a new computer or to fluorescent lights. Often these symptoms are not immediately recognized as being brought on by electromagnetic field exposure.

Five Common Symptoms of Electromagnetic Exposure
- Skin itch/rash
- Flushing/burning and/or tingling
- Memory loss
- Fatigue/weakness
- Headache
- Chest pain/heart problems

Other Symptoms of Electromagnetic Hypersensitivity Syndrome

Abnormal behavior	Inability to concentrate
Breathing difficulty	Irritability
Buzzing or ringing in ears	Mood swings
Chronic fatigue	Muscle and skeletal pains
Confusion	Muscular weakness
Cramps	Poor memory
Depression	Skin numbness
Dizziness	Sleep disturbances
Eye irritation	Stomach aches
Fainting	Weakening of hands and joints
Flu-like conditions	

The Chemical Connection

Multiple chemical sensitivity appears to predispose individuals to electromagnetic sensitivity or make them more susceptible to adverse effects of electromagnetic radiation. People with known chemical sensitivities have subsequently become electricity sensitive. In addition, a link has been observed in that the symptoms of multiple chemical exposure create essentially the same set of symptoms as exposure to electromagnetic fields. Both disorders share the same general involvement of the central nervous system and the immune system, producing virtually identical symptoms. It has been reported that up to 80% of chemically sensitive individuals are electromagnetic sensitive.

A possible explanation for this link is presented in the following example. Many individuals have reported acute exposure to pesticides just prior to becoming sensitive to electromagnetic fields. Organophosphate pesticide exposure is known to inhibit the function of an enzyme called cholinesterase, which is needed to prevent the accumulation of the neurotransmitter acetylcholine.

By inhibiting cholinesterase, the organophosphate pesticides in effect cause an excess of acetylcholine, which overstimulates the nervous system, producing symptoms. The connecting link with electromagnetic sensitivity comes from Russian research. Russian scientists have consistently found that when humans are exposed to microwave frequency radiation, the enzyme cholinesterase is again inhibited causing an excess of acetylcholine, and producing similar symptoms as in the pesticide studies.

This demonstrates how the same nervous system dysfunction can occur after chemical (pesticide) exposure as well as to radiation exposure. That radiation exposure can produce the same effect as a chemical poison in the body provides evidence for a radiation poisoning effect.

Limiting Exposure

Because of the amount of time spent in the bedroom, it is particularly important to decrease exposure in this area. Electric cords connecting appliances to the wall outlet can generate electrical fields even though the appliance has been switched off. Electric blankets, bedroom televisions, digital clocks, and bedside telephones may all increase exposure. Hidden wires in walls may generate electrical fields. Magnetic fields are capable of penetrating through walls, floors and ceilings.

Some individuals have experienced symptoms from televisions next to the wall in an adjoining room. More restful sleep is obtained by moving or eliminating all electrical devices and wiring in the immediate area. Remove or unplug all electrical appliances and keep them at least four feet from the bed.

In addition, authorities recommend the following. Practice prudent avoidance with digital clocks, electric blankets, water bed heaters, electric heating pads, fluorescent lights, halogen and high-intensity reading lights, and metal lamps. Use a deep bookcase headboard on the bed to increase distance from wiring in the wall. Another option is to buy a remote breaker cut-off switch that can turn off your bedroom electricity from anywhere in the house. Make sure that the head of the bed is not on the other side of the wall from the back of a TV, computer monitor, refrigerator or metal pipes as the magnetic field can go right through the wall.

The different fields that surround computer monitors, keyboards, computers and cables can be areas of substantial exposure because of the amount of time spent in close proximity to them. Visual display terminals emit several types of electromagnetic radiation: electrostatic field, electrical and magnetic alternating fields and radio frequency emissions.

The question of cellular phone safety has been raised since about 1993 by scientists and others who are concerned about the effect of the radiation emitted from these phones. Cases of brain cancer and other cancers have been reported. Laboratory studies have been performed with mixed findings. Researchers at Integrated Laboratory Systems, N.C. found that high levels of cellular phone radiation can cause chromosomal abnormalities in human blood cells.

A Swedish study concluded that cellular phones posed no increased risk for brain tumors, but in a very small group, tumors were more likely to be found on the side of the head where the phone was used. Over 100 million cellular phones are now in use in the United States.

It is important to become aware of the sources and cumulative effects of radiation exposure, particularly if your body is already compromised and exhibiting signs of chronic disease or allergy. Limiting sources of pollution of all types helps increase the immune system's power to combat illness. While you cannot eliminate all the sources of electropollution in today's world, you can take steps to limit your exposure.

Ways to Reduce the Effects of Electromagnetic Fields

1. Sit at least four to six feet away from the television set and limit the time in front of it.
2. Stay at least four feet away from microwave ovens in use and limit exposure time, or do not use them. Do not let children stand and watch food cook.
3. Obtain full spectrum lighting for fluorescent lights. Russian scientists report that full spectrum lights increase the body's tolerance to environmental pollutants.

4. Avoid buying a home near high-tension power lines or a microwave tower.

5. Use cellular phones as little as possible. The newer digital phones apparently emit less radiation than the older analog phones.

6. Stay at least a good arm length from you computer monitor.

7. Locate breaker boxes and where high-tension wires come into your house and avoid spending time near them.

8. Buy cars without computer components.

9. Use special transparent screens for electrical field grounding and glare reduction on your computer monitor.

10. Discuss radiation exposure with your doctor prior to having diagnostic X-rays taken. Request the minimum number of views necessary.

11. Avoid living near a nuclear power station, or next to a nuclear disposal site.

12. Avoid products containing radio-luminous dials and markers.

13. Avoid eyeglass lenses that contain uranium or thorium to enhance optical quality. Studies show these eyeglasses emit one millirad per hour.

Exposure to radiation from any source is an additional stress to the body, especially to its electromagnetic fields. It is best to limit exposure by becoming aware of the sources of radiation in the environment. By removing unnecessary stressors from the environment, a person suffering from allergic problems will respond to treatment more rapidly.

19

Seven Steps to Health

Allergy is the result of toxicity from all sources including chronic infections, deficiencies (primarily of enzymes, vitamins and minerals), and chronic digestive conditions. The consequences of these conditions are vastly under-recognized by most health professionals.

The Pottenger cat studies clearly demonstrate that allergy can be produced at will through diet in one to three generations of cats, and also reversed in one to three generations of cats through improved diet. Poor digestion of food is a precursor to a great deal of allergy. So many people create a compromised digestive tract by putting too much processed, heat-treated and chemicalized food into their systems when no proof exists that humans are able to digest it. Therefore, the body must make changes and adaptations in order to survive.

How is This Program Different?

Most books on allergy advise an elimination diet, in which you eliminate the allergenic foods for months or years. Other books encourage you to become a super sleuth and track down hidden food allergies, looking for fragments of chemicals and microscopic ingredients which can be hidden in your meals, your house or your environment. Still other books recommend that you rotate your foods, eating the same food only once every four or five days, or keeping a diet diary of everything you eat. While all these methods are good advice to help control allergies, they do not make you well to the point where you stay well. They are good methods only for as long as you continue to follow them.

A more effective approach to allergy recognizes the source or underlying conditions that produce it. The following program addresses the three most common underlying conditions seen in allergic individuals. It is important to work to correct all three conditions at the same time. This is an extremely important point because if only one of the underlying conditions is corrected, the other two conditions will continue to damage the body tissues and produce symptoms. When you have allergies, you have chronic infections, enzyme deficiencies, and poor digestive ability. All of the steps to wellness must be done together for effective results.

The amount of treatment required to reverse these conditions depends on the severity and duration of the allergies and the strength of the body's immune system. Four to six weeks is the average time required to turn the degenerative processes around and to allow for tissue healing.

Persons with mild allergic conditions respond faster than those with severe symptoms. This is because the treatment process must be administered more slowly in acutely ill persons. Following is a basic program that has worked with wonderful success on thousands of patients.

The Seven Healing Steps
1. Prepare the body to get well.
2. Eliminate allergens.
3. Enzyme therapy.
4. Build the immune system.
5. Professional care.
6. Healing techniques and dietary follow-up.
7. Think wellness and wholeness.

Step One
Prepare the Body to Get Well
Preparing the body means lowering the allergic or toxic load. Check your environment and eliminate sources of toxins, molds and fungi. Inspect gas stoves and furnaces to ensure there are no fumes or leaks. Use earth-friendly, less toxic household cleaners, cosmetics and personal care products. Avoid exposure to radiation.

Obtain a pure, clean source of water. Tap water is not recommended. Reverse osmosis or distilled water is preferable. The quality of bottled water can be difficult to determine. Before drinking bottled water, you should check with the company as to source of the water, content and quality.

Next, it is helpful to clean out the body. A fresh fruit and vegetable juice diet for three to ten days is desirable. This juice diet is not absolutely essential to the program, but it does lower the toxic load of the body and speeds up the healing process. It requires that you obtain a good juicer and use only fresh, preferably organically grown, raw fruits and vegetables. Health food stores carry good books on how to prepare juice, complete with many juice recipes.

Eliminate Infections: A big source of toxicity is infection by invading organisms such as yeast, fungi and parasites. Allergic individuals tend to have a high incidence of such infections, as they underlie the allergic condition. The organisms constitute a major source of toxicity and stress to the immune system, while the victim is often unaware of their presence. In order to regain health, these infections and infestations, if present, must be recognized and brought under control.

Candidiasis has come to the forefront because of increased publicity in recent years. It is more likely to be recognized than other infestations or infections by organisms. There are many good therapies for candidiasis. Some programs, however, work faster than others do and some are only temporarily effective. It is not uncommon for the afflicted individual to be on a Candida diet for months and still not be restored to health. Another problem commonly seen is the removal of foods from the diet for such a lengthy time that the body 's nutritional state can be compromised. In some cases, the patient becomes anxious and fanatical about foods in general - another undesirable state.

A sensible program of diet, nutrients and an understanding of the goals will bring Candida under control in a short time. Since Candida is a normal inhabitant of the intestine, the goal is not to kill it off completely. The goal is to bring its numbers back in balance with the other normal residents of the colon, and then to keep them in line by increasing the general health of the person and his immune system.

An effective anti-fungal (Candida) program consists of three parts:
1. Use an anti-fungal agent and acidophilus to reculture the colon.
2. Eliminate all forms of sugar and any irritating and intolerant foods.
3. Take enzymes to ensure the proper breakdown of foods

While there are prescription anti-fungal agents available from medical doctors, there are also many effective anti-fungal formulas that you can obtain on your own from the health food store. In general, a formula which includes one or more anti-fungal agents is most effective. These days, most good health food stores will carry one or more anti-fungal formulas.

Active anti-fungal agents that work to eliminate Candida include the following:

Biotin	Garlic
Caprylic acid	Grapefruit seed extract

A good product will combine one or more of the above in a formula with other herbs and vitamins. For best results, the formula must be taken for 4 to 6 weeks.

In addition to the anti-fungal formula, supplementation with probiotics (lactobacillus acidophilus and bifidus) is necessary to reculture the intestine and prevent the Candida from overgrowing again. Select a good quality acidophilus and bifidus formula from the refrigerator of the health food store. Check the expiry date on the bottle. Probiotics are live organisms whose activity decreases with time and exposure to heat.

Eliminate all sugar products and any foods which you know you do not digest well or produce a reaction of any sort. In general, most vegetables have anti-fungal effects. Therefore, a diet high in vegetable products is recommended. Steaming vegetables helps increase their digestibility by breaking down fiber, but of course, also destroys enzymes. Steam vegetables only when necessary. Fresh vegetable juice is a good alternative.

Sugar is in many packaged foods, so read the labels. Sugar helps feed the Candida organism and encourages its growth, so its elimination during the course of anti-fungal therapy is absolutely necessary.

Candida Reduction Program

This program has proven successful because it is quickly effective without being overly restrictive, which leads to excellent patient compliance. In order to diminish the number of Candida organisms, combine a formula similar to this one.

Caprylic acid	300 mg
Sorbic Acid (Potassium Sorbate)	100 mg

Propionic Acid (Calcium Propionate)	100 mg
Biotin	300 mcg
Vitamin E (d-Alpha Tocopherol)	5 IU

In adults, a recommended dosage is one to two capsules three times daily. Caprylic acid, along with a variety of fatty acids and biotin is known to be effective in the control of Candida albicans and other yeast or fungal infections. At the same time, take a good quality Lactobacillus acidophilus (probiotic) supplement.

When a formula such as the above is used, the diet does not have to be unduly strict. Only the worst offending foods are eliminated and only for four to six weeks. Almost everyone will respond in this period of time. If a person does not respond, either the products chosen are not of good quality or the person is not following the program for the prescribed time.

The Candida (anti-fungal) diet must be followed for four to six weeks.

Water

Yeast products often react allergically in the body when Candida is present, which is why exclusion of all yeast products is necessary. Drink six to eight glasses of pure water each day. There will be toxins and waste products formed as Candida breaks down and is eliminated. The water aids in this process by diluting the toxins, preventing discomforts that might otherwise occur. Symptoms that indicate you are not drinking enough water at this time include headaches, chills, fever, muscle aches and rashes.

Candida (Anti-fungal) Diet
Foods You Can Eat
Vegetables

Asparagus	Lettuce
Beet	Onion
Broccoli	Parsley
Brussels sprouts	Parsnip
Cabbage	Peas
Carrot	Potato
Cauliflower	Radish
Celery	Squash

Cucumber	Sweet potato
Eggplant	Tomato
Green Pepper	Zucchini

Fruits

(Note: Limit fruit to two whole, fresh fruits per day. Do not use fruit juice.)

Apple	Nectarine
Apricot	Orange
Banana	Papaya
Berries	Peach
Cherry	Pear
Grape	Pineapple
Grapefruit	Plum
Mango	

Whole grains–all kinds

Unleavened bread, all flours except wheat (no yeast)

Unfermented protein foods

Seeds and nuts–all kinds except peanuts

Fats–Butter or extra virgin olive oil for cooking.

Olive oil contains oleic acid, which has been shown to hinder the conversion of Candida albicans to the more harmful mycelia fungal form.

Foods You Must Avoid

All types of sugar and sugar-containing foods

Fermented products

Most packaged and processed foods (Check labels for sugar and yeast.)

Alcoholic beverages including beer and wine

Baked goods–cookies, cakes, pies

Breads and all products containing yeast

Cheese

Dairy products–all, except butter

Fruits–dried and candied

Ice cream

Meats–processed and smoked meats (cold cuts)

Mushrooms
Peanuts
Sugary beverages–all fruit juices, soft drinks, soda pop, diet soda
Vinegar-containing foods
Yogurt

Parasites

Many parasites are cyclic, going through dormant and active phases, which means that they cannot always be found by testing. If suspected, the tests should be performed several times in order to rule out the presence of these organisms.

When parasites are present, herbal formulas will help to eliminate them. Formulas containing black walnut, pumpkin seeds, Artemesia annua (wormwood), garlic and cloves have been effective. Many good formulas containing several herbs are available at health food stores. The formula should be taken continuously for a minimum of 30 days since it is important to interrupt the life cycle of the parasite from its cyst (dormant) stage to its larva (active) stage.

Healing the Intestine

A herbal formula that is extremely helpful for healing the lining of the digestive tract is a liquid containing artichoke, dandelion and ten other herbs. It will produce noticeable healing changes very rapidly, usually within three days. The ten other herbs are turmeric root, St. Mary's thistle, blessed thistle, buckbean leaves, milfoil herb, gentian root, wormwood, calamus root, chamomile and fennel. Good quality liquid chlorophyll is also beneficial.

Other green supplement products including: chlorella, spirulina, and blue-green algae are loaded with carotenoids, enzymes, and many trace nutrients and can contribute to healing the digestive tract.

Glutamine is an amino acid that helps heal the cells that line the small intestine and stomach and it is the principal source of energy for those cells. Glutamine can probably help heal the intestinal lining more effectively than any other single nutrient.

Three other herbs that promote intestinal healing include licorice in its deglycyrrhizinated form, chamomile and marshmallow. Deglycyrrhiz-

241

inated licorice is known to soothe inflamed mucous membranes in the digestive tract and increase the production of mucin, which protects the lining of the intestine. It also has antibiotic and antioxidant properties. The deglycyrrhizinated form has had the portion of the licorice root associated with increasing blood pressure and water retention removed and the mucous membrane- healing part of the root retained.

Chamomile tea is also soothing to inflamed and irritated mucous membranes and is high in a bioflavonoid called apigenin. Marshmallow root is a traditional remedy for irritated and inflamed mucous membranes in the digestive tract.

To summarize, step 1 of allergy elimination

1. Take herbal and nutrient formulas to either diminish the number, or destroy the pathogenic organisms.
2. Reculture the bowel using probiotic supplements.
3. Repair tissues by diminishing food and chemical stresses and taking herbal and nutrient healing supplements.

When organisms such as Candida and other parasites are eliminated or brought under control, it is not unusual for 80% of the allergies displayed by the patient to be improved in just four to six weeks on the above program.

Step Two
Eliminate Allergens.

Eliminate the main food allergens for the first four to six weeks. If you do not know to what you are allergic or sensitive, you have two choices.

1. Eliminate the most common allergens such as dairy products, especially milk and cheese, wheat, eggs, corn, peanuts, beef and pork and all obvious chemicals in your environment.
2. Consult one of the doctors from the referral directory in the Resources section of this book.

On an effective program, foods are temporarily eliminated in order to give the digestive and immune systems time to recover and heal. After four to six weeks the foods can be reintroduced one at a time. Reinstate only healthy foods. Do not reinstate homogenized, pasteurized milk, processed packaged foods, or sugary foods.

Step Three
Enzyme Therapy

Nutritional enzyme therapy is the cornerstone of effective allergy treatment. This safe and non-toxic therapy has one major advantage; it has the power to eliminate allergies. Information on enzyme therapy has greatly increased in the last few years. Effective plant enzymes contain the enzymes protease, amylase, lipase and cellulase. Many enzyme formulas may list additional enzymes and herbs, but these should be the first four enzymes at the top of the ingredient list.

Nutritional plant enzymes have a wide range of activity, work throughout the intestine, and ensure the proper breakdown of foods in a compromised digestive tract. When foods are fully digested, they are basically rendered non-allergic. In addition, the enzyme cellulase has been shown to digest microorganisms such as fungi/yeasts, which includes Candida albicans. In the clinical setting plant enzymes have proven to be a quick and efficient way to restore health from allergies.

For our purposes, there are three categories of therapeutic enzymes - nutritional plant enzymes, pancreatic enzymes, and antioxidant enzymes.

Nutritional Plant Enzymes: These are enzymes taken from plants under low heat conditions and concentrated. They contain protease, amylase, lipase and cellulase. They are the only enzymes capable of working both in the stomach and the small intestine as they are active at a pH range of approximately 3 to 9. After ingestion of food, they help the digestive process for up to an hour before the stomach pH finally falls below 3. Later, they are reactivated in the alkaline pH of the small intestine and help to complete the process of digestion.

When plant enzymes are given between meals, instead of being used to digest food, a portion of them is absorbed intact into the blood stream and supports the work of the metabolic enzymes, especially those involved in immune processes.

Protease helps the immune system by digesting bacteria, parasites, partially digested protein particles and other toxins. It is also capable of playing a role in neutralizing inflammations. The enzymes amylase and lipase play a part in digesting some viruses as well as healing allergic eruptions of the skin.

Other food enzymes, such as bromelain and papain, although useful in some conditions, work best in a temperature range much higher than that of the human body. This is one reason why nutritional plant enzymes are preferable.

Antioxidant Enzymes: These enzymes are not used to digest food. Instead, they convert damaging free radicals to oxygen and water, rendering them harmless to the body. They help protect the body from the effects of ionizing radiation and rancid fats.

Antioxidant enzymes also appear to participate in breaking apart immune complexes lodged in the body as a result of allergic reactions. Thus, they also help to reduce inflammation in the tissues.

Antioxidant enzymes are produced from plants, mostly sprouts, under a low heat process. The main antioxidant enzymes found in capsules are superoxide dismutase, catalase, glutathione peroxidase and methionine reductase.

How Much and What Type Should I Take?

The types and amounts of enzymes needed in allergic conditions depend upon the severity of the allergy. An average program would supplement two capsules of nutritional plant enzymes before each meal. Two or more capsules of pancreatin can be given after meals when inflammation or pain is present. Pancreatic enzyme therapy is effective in controlling pain reactions from kinin-mediated inflammation that sometimes develops in the intestine usually from 15 minutes to two hours after the meal.

Nutritional plant enzymes help in the healing of the intestines and normalization of digestive function in several ways:

1. They ensure proper digestion of food.

2. They take stress off the digestive organs and allow them to rest.

3. They prevent further allergic reactions, which can damage the intestinal tissue.

Step Four
Build the Immune System

Taking a nutrient formula to build the immune system helps speed up healing. A good immune building formula will contain vitamins A, C and E, minerals such as zinc and selenium, glandulars such as thymus (bovine) and lymph (bovine) and herbs such as echinacea. Especially with Candida overgrowth the tissue content of vitamin A is often low. Other herbs and nutrients which help support the immune system include: goldenseal, garlic, astragulus, wild indigo, myrrh, boneset, bioflavonoids, beta carotene, B-6, glutathione, coenzyme Q-10, spleen (bovine), and colostrum. A good multiple vitamin and mineral supplement is also recommended.

Step Five
Professional Care

Many forms of chiropractic adjustment techniques not only work to correct structural and neurological dysfunction, but some types of non-force adjusting appear to correct the energetic balance of the body as well. The result is a better-integrated functioning of the body as a whole.

Chiropractors using these techniques are often helpful in recommending appropriate nutritional supplements and enzymes. For severe allergic conditions, professional help is recommended. You may obtain a referral through the directory listed under Resources

Step Six:
Healing Techniques and Dietary Follow-up

Homeopathy: Desensitization and neutralization of allergy is frequently assisted by the use of homeopathic preparations, which are minute dilutions of specific substances. These preparations, in liquid or tablet form, are generally taken under the tongue. These remedies are completely safe and easy to administer. Coffee should not be taken when the allergic individual is under treatment, as it can interfere with the action of the homeopathic preparation.

Homeopathic remedies work well on all types of allergy. They are helpful with food allergens as well as with airborne allergens such as: dust, pollen, grass and mold, and with allergies, to dogs, cats and horses. They can be added into the program from the start or at any other time. Their action appears to be increased after the allergic individual is detoxified. For this reason, they are useful for allergies, which are still active after Candida, and parasites are under control and the digestive tract has had time to heal.

However, particularly for airborne allergies and Candida, they can be very helpful from the start of the program.

Inhalation Therapy: It is interesting to note that many inhalant allergies are eliminated when proper diet, accompanied by an improvement indigestion and enzyme therapy, are employed. On occasions when improvement does not occur, as expected, there is special help for stubborn inhalant allergies. When sinus symptoms persist, fungus lodged in the sinuses is often the reason.

When fungus is present, tea-tree (Melaleuca) oil can be used to speed up healing. Put five to ten drops of tea-tree oil in a basin of hot water. Then, breathing through the nose, inhale the steam deeply and expel through the mouth. This should be done twice daily for three days. Four to five breaths at a time are sufficient. Tea tree oil comes from Australia, where there are over three hundred known species of tea trees. It has gained popularity recently for its anti-fungal properties.

Dietary Follow-Up: Except for the severest cases, the allergic individual should be symptom-free in approximately six weeks when the first six steps have been followed. Damaged tissues may still be healing, however, so precautions should be taken.

If a person returns to his old habits, old problems tend to come back. Once a person is allergy-free, he generally does not want to do things that will cause a return of the condition.

After returning the healthful foods to the diet, the person should continue to take plant enzymes before meals, especially when cooked foods are consumed. This supplies the missing enzymes from those foods and helps to keep digestion competent. The only other supplement that may be needed is a good vitamin and mineral formula, again, because foods tend to be lacking in nutrients. A diet of 70% fresh raw fruits, vegetables, seeds and nuts and 30% grains, eggs and protein foods is recommended to prevent the return of allergy.

Step Seven
Think Wellness and Wholeness.

No allergy program would be complete without focusing attention on the importance of the body-mind connection. When allergy arises, it is easy to view the world as a hostile place where hidden dangers lurk. One can become anxious and wary about all sorts of environmental toxins and food ingredients in a supreme effort to protect oneself. While increased awareness of these matters is often necessary to recover from allergy, over-concern is not.

You cannot avoid all environmental poisons and food toxins. Therefore, avoid the "big stuff." Your new knowledge has increased your awareness of major sources of toxicity so that you may now choose to eliminate them from your environment. In doing so, you unburden your healing system. A normal, healthy person is not overly concerned with each chemical he comes in contact with: his body automatically neutralizes and eliminates these chemicals when his tolerance level is not exceeded. Thus, no symptoms occur.

When you have followed the first six steps for six weeks, your body is on a healing course. The minute amount of allergen that once created agonizing symptoms will no longer have that power. Your tolerance will have increased and will continue to increase until your body has normalized and healed.

Once you have put the healing steps in motion and have established the habits necessary to carry them out, it is time to mentally relax. Anxiety itself is known to block healing. If you are experiencing anxiety, depression or any other negative feeling, deliberately think of a happy or positive thought. While you think this positive thought, your brain will begin to produce hormones, which will bring forth the feeling. Rest assured that your body now has what it needs to continue healing to the normal state.

Mentally, allergy no longer concerns you. It is time to stop thinking about allergy and to think only wellness and wholeness. Each day becomes a new discovery of your body's increased ability to deal with its environment. Discovery of these new strengths feeds your excitement and adds to your belief that you are whole and well. As you continue your thoughts of wholeness and wellness, your beliefs become knowing.

The *Seven Steps* are a basic program for the average person with allergies. In more severe cases, professional care is advised as there are many specialized alternate therapies that may speed the course of healing. Also, if you suspect allergies, or do not know the cause of your symptoms, or do not know to what you are allergic, you should seek professional advice. This is especially true when parasites are present as they can be difficult to detect.

Another reason for seeking outside help is to determine your individual nutrient requirements. In the hundreds of cases of allergy I have treated, no two have been identical, and no two programs have been exactly the same. All, however, have revolved around the basic program of detoxification; checking for pathological organisms; enzyme therapy; nutrients to build the immune system, and normalizing the nerve and energetic pathways of the body.

Additional Nutritional Considerations

Food Combining: Most people with allergy have a compromised digestive tract, whether they are aware of it or not. Even when no symptoms in the digestive area are apparent, the ability to digest food is often inadequate, causing allergic symptoms to arise in other areas of the body. Properly combined food takes stress off the digestive tract and allows for more efficient digestion. When food is digested completely, the particles do not become allergens.

Properly combined food requires less enzymes for digestion. In an allergic person, the vital function of enzyme production is compromised. When food is combined properly, less stress is imposed on the digestive tract allowing it time to recover and again function optimally. Enzyme stores then have a chance to build up, and improved digestion prevents allergic reactions from taking place.

There are many food combining charts available on the market today. Many are very complex, explaining the ideal combining methods. In severe allergic cases, this is helpful. However, for the average person with allergies, a modified combining method is sufficient. Here are the most important points of proper food combining, which have worked well in hundreds of clinical cases of allergy, are.

1. Eat all fruit alone, without any other type of food for at least one hour before and one hour after ingestion of the fruit.

2. Protein foods can be eaten with any vegetables except the starchy ones such as potato, yam and corn.

3. Whole grains can be eaten with any kind of vegetable including starchy ones.

4. Never follow a protein meal with any kind of sugar dessert, including fruit. When these are eaten together, they cannot be digested thoroughly. This invites not only allergic reactions, but toxins are formed in the intestines which can then be absorbed, stressing the liver and immune system.

Nutritional Deficiencies: Nutrition and allergy interact in several ways. Some individuals may have trouble meeting all their nutritional requirements because they have been forced to eliminate many foods (their allergenic foods) from their diet. Also, since people with food allergies have digestive enzyme problems, they have difficulty breaking down and digesting certain foods. They thereby fail to obtain the nutrients they need.

Some people with allergic problems have special individual biochemical requirements for more of certain vitamins and minerals. Continued allergic stresses on the biochemical system nearly always cause nutritional imbalances or deficiencies. There are many nutrients which benefit allergy. Certainly all of the nutrients known to support the immune system are helpful in allergic conditions.

Key Nutrients Known to Support the Immune System

Vitamin C: Vitamin C appears to act as a natural antihistamine. Large doses of eight grams or more have been known to break an allergic reaction in four to five hours.

Researchers at the Methodist Hospital in Brooklyn studied four hundred people with blood levels low in vitamin C and high in histamine. These people were given 1,000 mg of vitamin C daily. It was found that the histamine levels of the blood dropped, and improvement was seen in the allergic symptoms.

Citrus Bioflavonoids: Citrus bioflavonoids, which are actually part of a complete vitamin C, enhance its utilization. Studies done on animals have shown that citrus bioflavonoids may favorably alter the body's metabolism of vitamin C, raising the concentration of the nutrient in certain tissues and enhancing its availability to the body.

The bioflavonoid curcumin appears to have greater anti-inflammatory action than cortisone. Another bioflavonoid, quercitin, pre-

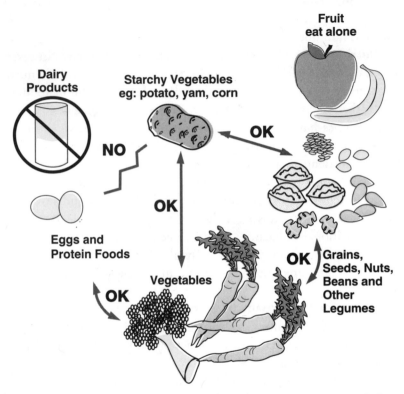

Fruit
eat alone

Dairy
Products

Starchy Vegetables
eg: potato, yam, corn

NO

OK

OK

Eggs and
Protein Foods

Vegetables

OK

OK } Grains,
Seeds, Nuts,
Beans and
Other
Legumes

1. *Eat protein with non-starchy vegetables*
2. *Eat vegetables with grains, seeds, nuts and legumes*
3. *Eat fruit alone.*

4. *Dairy products are not recommended. If eaten, dairy products are in protein group and combine with vegetables only.*
5. *Sweetened desserts not recommended – especially should not follow after protein meal*

Figure 7. **Food Combining**

vents the formation of the inflammatory leukotrienes. It also reduces the release of histamine.

Even though vitamin C and the bioflavonoids are discussed separately, best results are obtained when they are used together as nature intended.

Vitamin C works more effectively when accompanied by B-complex vitamins, especially pantothenic acid. Without adequate amounts of pantothenic acid, the adrenal hormone cortisone cannot be produced. Natural cortisone relieves and lessens the duration of the allergic reactions.

B6: Another vitamin known to have antihistamine effects is vitamin B6, which is extremely important to numerous enzyme systems in the body. As little as 2.5 mg is enough under most circumstances to achieve an anti-histamine effect. Raw liver capsules or tablets also exert an anti-histamine effect on the body.

Essential Fatty Acids: The essential fatty acids, LA and LNA, are known powerful inhibitors of inflammation. This is because they are essential for the production of prostaglandins, which in turn regulate inflammation. Of these, fresh pressed, unrefined flaxseed oil is probably the best choice. Flaxseed oil contains the highest proportion of Omega 3 and also contains some Omega 6. Fish oil is a good source of Omega 3 in the form of EPA. However, flaxseed oil has the advantages of being better tasting, from a vegetable source and less expensive, and not containing toxins often found in fish.

GLA (gamma-linoleic acid) from evening primrose oil is another nutrient that inhibits the inflammatory response. It has been shown to be effective for people with a history of allergy and eczema.

EPA (eicosapentaenoic acid) from DHA-rich microalgae displaces arachidonic acid in the cell membranes, leaving less arachidonic acid available for inflammatory reactions.

Minerals: Minerals are necessary to build enzyme systems. Three minerals especially important to the allergic individual are zinc, selenium and magnesium.

Zinc is perhaps the most vital immune mineral. Without enough zinc, many of the lymph tissues actually shrink, including the thymus and the lymph nodes. The concentration of zinc in the cells affects how energetically the white blood cells attack invaders. Studies show how low zinc levels reduce the number of T-cells. Zinc is important in skin problems and for immune system integrity. When combined with vitamins A, C and E and essential fatty acids, zinc can help speed the healing of eczema.

More recently, research has uncovered the connection of zinc to essential fatty acid metabolism, demonstrating zinc to be crucial to the conversion of some of the nutritionally-derived, essential fatty acids to their active form.

Deficiency of selenium results in diminished resistance to all types of infection, lowered antibody formation and reduced ability of the immune system T-cells to destroy foreign invaders. Supplementation with selenium has been shown to reverse these problems.

Magnesium participates in numerous reactions related to the competence of the immune system, including growth and transformation of B-lymphocytes and the process of protein synthesis whereby immunoglobulins are formed. In clinical studies, magnesium is frequently found to be deficient in allergic individuals.

Vitamin A: A lack of vitamin A will cause atrophic changes (wasting away) in the thymus gland and spleen. Vitamin A acts to eliminate free radicals before they can do severe cell damage, thus strengthening the immune system.

Researchers have found that children with low vitamin A had abnormally low levels of T-cells in their blood. Vitamin A makes T-cells more active and stronger.

Vitamin E

Physicians at Cornell University have demonstrated that vitamin E stimulates antibody production. It helps the T-cells to react faster and more strongly, increasing resistance to disease. As an antioxidant, vitamin E is capable of deactivating free radicals before they can destroy cells.

There are over fifty crucial immune nutrients, and they must be in precise balance for the immune system to work powerfully and efficiently. It is important when considering nutritional needs to recognize each person's inborn biochemical individuality. Every person has a metabolic pattern all his own, which increases or decreases the need for specific vitamins and minerals. Typically, nutrients are not like medicines directed at specific diseases. Instead, they work together synergistically to promote a healthy metabolism.

20

Frequently Asked Questions

Q. *Why do I have so many symptoms and my medical tests*
are normal?
Answer: It is matter of degree. Disease begins with small alterations in body chemistry or function. These tiny, insidious changes usually go undetected while the body's tissues attempt to make the necessary corrections. When the body's ability to compensate for these changes is exhausted, more changes occur which alter normal body physiology. At this point, noticeable symptoms occur but usually not physical findings.

However, when this process continues uncorrected, it eventually results in changes in tissue or structure that can now be found on medical tests and diagnosed as disease or pathology. In other words, symptoms must progress to a certain point before they will show on a medical exam.

Q. *After I have eliminated allergic or intolerant foods for four*
to six weeks, how do I start adding them back into the diet?
Answer: When you have followed the complete program and are feeling better, your intestine will have had time to heal. People do not always realize the healthy internal changes that have taken place during the four to six weeks. The intestine will not be in the same malfunctioning state as when you started the program because you have removed several causes that contributed to the incompetent intestine.

You begin to add foods back into the diet one at a time leaving a day or two in between. Begin with any vegetables that were eliminated, then add in fruits. Protein foods may be added next, fol-

255

lowed by grains. Do not be in a hurry to add wheat back into the diet. Hopefully you have had time to experiment with many other types of grains during the four to six weeks and will continue to use some of them. Wheat can be eaten conservatively, but do not make it the only grain that you eat. Sugars (desserts) and homogenized, pasteurized milk cannot be recommended to be reintroduced into the diet. Small quantities are sometimes tolerated but this is very individual.

Q: *Are there any healthy dairy products that can be used when homogenized, pasteurized milk is withdrawn from the diet?*

Answer: When a person is allergic or intolerant to milk, it is important to eliminate all dairy products for a minimum of six weeks (although it is often wise to wait eight weeks or longer), in order to give the body time to heal, and for the milk antibodies to have time to leave the system.,

Once health is restored, there are healthy milk products that often can be utilized if desired. Yogurt is a fermented milk product with enhanced digestibility because it is virtually predigested by the friendly fermentation bacteria, rendering its nutrients including calcium more bioavailable. Quality yogurt, usually obtained from a health food store, contains live and active cultures. These living cultures have been destroyed in many supermarket brands and this product can no longer be considered a true yogurt and its primary health benefits have been lost.

The vast majority of adults do not produce the enzyme lactase, which digests lactose, the sugar in milk. Active, live lactobacilli such as L.acidophilus and L.bulgaricus supply the enzyme lactase, which makes a milk product more digestible. The protein in yogurt is less allergenic than in milk since the lactic acid action increases protein digestibility by rendering the protein into smaller particles such as peptides and free amino acids.

Another product used for thousands of years but not well known in North America is kefir, a fermented milk that is a traditional food in many parts of the world. With kefir's long history of health-enhancing qualities, it has some advantages over yogurt. Kefir is even easier to digest than yogurt and the kefir culture (live microorganisms) is hardier, and will self-generate more easily that yogurt culture.

Milk used to make kefir does not have to be preheated like milk used for making yogurt. Kefir contains smaller curds than yogurt, and active enzymes which increases its digestibility. Along with its living micro-organisms, kefir is also rich in proteins, minerals and vitamins. According to Dr. Orla-Jenson, a Danish bacteriologist, "Kefir digests yeast cells and has a beneficial effect on intestinal flora."

Butter can almost always be used at any time on the program covered in this book. Fresh, organic, unsalted butter is the type recommended. If any type of reaction occurs when a dairy product (even a healthy one) is reintroduced into the diet, it must be discontinued for at least another two to four weeks before being tried again.

Q **• Are you saying that I should never eat any cooked food • again?**

Answer: I am not recommending that you should never eat any cooked food. I am emphasizing the role of raw food in the natural diet. It is important to realize what the differences are between raw and cooked foods, an important one being enzyme content. Since adequate enzyme levels help protect the body from allergic reactions, enzymes become especially important to allergic individuals. I have never had a patient who converted to a totally raw food diet. However, I have had hundreds of patients who have recovered from allergy.

By the same token, a raw food diet is not an extreme diet. The totally cooked food, processed food, radiated food, chemicalized food diet is actually the extreme diet, as no other people on the face of the earth have ever before existed on it and there is no scientific evidence that they can.

If your objective is to eliminate allergy and to stay well, strive for a balanced ratio between cooked and raw foods.

Changing the diet to 70% raw and 30% cooked food is adequate to meet this objective. Whenever you eat cooked food, replace those missing enzymes with nutritional plant enzyme supplements. When the enzyme content of the diet remains high, allergies will not return.

Q **• How much of the essential fatty acids LA (Omega 6) and • LNA (Omega 3) is required per day?**

Answer: While there are no RDAs for LA and LNA established at

257

this time, the fact that these two fatty acids are indispensable to health and life has been substantiated. Based on laboratory studies and other evidence, it is believed that the requirement for LA is 2% of daily calories eaten. This is six grams on a 2,500 calorie diet. The requirement for LNA is considered to be 1% of calories eaten or three grams per day. Approximately one tablespoon of flaxseed oil per day will supply enough LNA.

Although a lack of these nutrients results in disease, only small quantities are required to maintain health.

Q: *Why do you recommend flaxseed oil?*

Answer: Flaxseed oil is the highest source of LNA, containing between 50% and 60%. This is the essential fatty acid that is deficient in most western diets. In addition, flaxseed oil contains between 15% and 25% LA. This means that you can obtain both essential fatty acids from one oil.

The LNA from flaxseed oil incorporates itself into the membranes of the cells of the body and attracts oxygen to the cells. Besides oxygenating the cells, oxygen acts as a barrier to bacteria and viruses.

The whole seed of flax can be ground up and used to top cereals and salads. Flax seed contains all the essential amino acids making it a complete protein. It supplies many vitamins and trace minerals and is an excellent source of fiber.

Flax seed has historically been used to heal digestive ailments.

Inflammation of the stomach, intestines and colon have been helped as well as constipation.

Q: *How should nuts and seeds be eaten?*

Answer: Nuts and seeds should be eaten raw. However, they contain substances called enzyme inhibitors. These inhibitors stop the seeds from sprouting until conditions are appropriate. For example, wheat found in ancient Egyptian tombs has been sprouted in this century. Enzyme inhibitors are the source of much indigestion when nuts and seeds are eaten raw. In order to inactivate the enzyme inhibitors, seeds and nuts must either be sprouted or cooked. Cooking, however, destroys LA and LNA as well as many enzymes and nutrients.

Nuts and seeds are best soaked in pure water for 12 to 24 hours depending on the kind of seeds or nuts. After soaking, seeds and nuts will have up to twenty times their original enzyme content and the enzyme inhibitors will be inactivated.

Grains and beans are most easily digested when they have been soaked for 24 hours before cooking. Since these foods are usually prepared by cooking, they should be consumed in smaller quantities (part of the 30%) than raw foods, and the missing food enzymes should be supplemented.

Q: *If allergy is an inflammatory condition, why not just take anti-inflammatory drugs?*

Answer: All drugs have undesirable side effects when taken over weeks, months and years. It is better to normalize the underlying condition producing the inflammation.

The body produces its own inflammation fighters to combat allergic inflammation. These substances are proteases, pancreatin, cortisone and prostaglandins. The key is to stimulate your own body processes to produce these substances while simultaneously discouraging allergen/antibody reactions from occurring. The main tool you have to work with is diet.

Q: *I have too much acid in my stomach because my stomach burns whenever I eat. What can I do besides take antacids?*

Answer: Burning pain in the stomach is not necessarily a sign of too much acid in the stomach. Studies show that most people over the age of forty actually have too little stomach acid. Both conditions are known to create burning pain in the stomach.

While antacids do stop pain, they also contribute to other undesirable problems. Frequent taking of antacids alkalinizes the stomach, which is the only organ in the body that is supposed to be acid. This has the following effects:

1. It upsets normal mineral relationships in the body. For example, phosphorus becomes depleted in the blood when antacids

containing magnesium hydroxide or aluminum hydroxide are taken. Decreased phosphorus results in lowered absorption of calcium from the intestines.

2. It hinders absorption of calcium and other minerals, which require an acid medium for absorption.
3. It shuts down normal digestion in the stomach so that foods may leave the stomach in a partially digested form. Partially digested particles of food stress the pancreas, are absorbed through the intestine to create allergies, and may ferment or putrefy in the lower bowel to create toxins.
4. It stresses the pH balance of the body.

A better approach to alleviating burning stomach pain is the following:

1. Eliminate food allergens from the diet.
2. Eat whole fresh food in its natural form.
3. Use the rules of correct food combining.
4. Do not overeat.
5. Do not drink alcohol with meals.
6. Do not follow meals with sweet desserts.
7. Do not eat when sick or emotionally upset.
8. If burning pain occurs, look for the cause and supplement with plant enzymes. Two capsules of nutritional plant enzymes may be taken every fifteen minutes until the pain subsides.

Q. *Is frequent eating of small amounts of food throughout the day the best way to eat?*

Answer: Frequent eating of small quantities of food will relieve symptoms in some conditions such as hypoglycemia and digestive problems, but may not be the best way to eat for health. Studies with laboratory animals show that frequent eating uses more enzymes. Eating fewer times per day and less food altogether produces healthier animals with longer life spans.

21

Victory over Allergy

As we have seen, allergy is an inflammatory condition in the body. All inflammation comes from four sources: injury, infection, degeneration and allergy. No matter where inflammation occurs, it is all nearly identical. If the immune system can produce inflammation and allergy, then the immune system can also correct it.

To overcome allergy, increased awareness is the key.

1. Increase your awareness that allergy can be involved in your symptoms.
2. Increase your awareness that you have the power to take control of your health. No one knows your body better than you do.
3. Increase your awareness that faulty digestion is involved in allergy.
4. Increase your awareness of your body's electromagnetic properties.
5. Increase your awareness of enzymes and their important role in allergy.

Enzymes have been termed the rescue remedy for allergy because people notice very rapid changes for the better when nutritional plant enzymes are taken.

You do not recover from allergy by treating one part of the body or by simply eliminating histamine or by making yourself comfortable with medications. You treat allergy by normalizing body functions.

No doctor can give you health. Health is a precious gift you give yourself.

Sequence of Healing Events
natural food = normal digestion = normal biochemistry
= normal energy = normal health = normal body

Appendix 1

Foods That May Contain Sugar

Cakes	Honey
Candy bars	Ice cream
Canned fruit	Jams
Carbonated beverages	Jelly
Cereals	Maple sugar
Chocolates	Marmalade
Cookies	Milkshakes
Desserts (most)	Molasses
Doughnuts	Pastries
Fruit drinks	Raw sugar
Fruit juice	Soft drinks
Fruit juice concentrate	Sorghum
Fruit snacks	Syrup

Sugar is hidden in many products. Be sure to read labels. Here are some other names for sugar

Barley malt	Invert sugar
Brown sugar	Lactose
Caramel	Malt syrup
Corn syrup solids	Maltose
Corn syrup,	Mannitol
Demerara sugar	Maple syrup
Dextran	Rice syrup

263

Dextrose,	Sorbitol,
Fructose	Sucrose
Glucose	Turbinado sugar
Glucose solids	Xylitol
Golden sugar	Yellow sugar

Foods that May Contain Yeast

Beer	Hamburger buns
Breads	Hotdog buns
Brewer's yeast	Ketchup
Buttermilk	Mayonnaise
Cake	Mushrooms
Cake mixes	Pastries
Cheese (all kinds)	Rolls
Cookies	Vinegar
Cottage cheese	Wine
Crackers	

Bread-like Products that can be made Without Yeast

Baking powder biscuits	Rye bread
Muffins	(some types - read label)
Pancakes	Tortillas
Pita bread (read label)	

Foods That May Contain Wheat

Biscuits	Gravy
Bran flakes	Hamburger
Bread mixes	Hot cereals
Breaded meat	Ice cream cones
Breads, all kinds	Macaroni
Bulgur	Mixed meat dishes
Cakes	Muffins
Candy bars	Noodles
Cold cereals	Pancakes
Cookies	Pasta

Corn flakes
Couscous
Crackers
Doughnuts
Dumplings
Durum
Flours
Graham flour
Pumpernickel flour
Semolina flour
White flour
Whole wheat flour

Pies
Popovers
Pretzels
Puddings
Rolls
Rye bread
Sauces
Sausages
Soups
Spaghetti
Waffles
Wheat germ

There are many alternatives to wheat, although you may have to bake you own muffins and other products. Some tortillas and pita breads contain no wheat. Most health food stores carry bread baked without wheat. You can also purchase many types of excellent flours as alternatives to wheat including: rice flour, rye, barley, oat, millet, buckwheat, soy, and potato flours. Other wheat-free mixes are all available for making pancakes and other products. Ask health food store personnel to show you all the products they carry that do not contain wheat. Spelt and triticale are other alternatives.

Foods That May Contain Milk

Biscuits
Buttermilk
Cakes
Candies
Cheeses
Chocolate
Chowder
Cocoa drinks
Coffee whiteners
Cookies
Cream pies
Cream sauces
Creamed foods

Hot cakes
Hot chocolate mixes
Ice cream
Junket
Malted milk
Margarine
Mashed potatoes
Milk chocolate
Muffins
Omelets
Pastries
Salad dressings
Scalloped dishes

Custards	Scrambled eggs
Doughnuts	Sherbet
Foods prepared au gratin	Soufflés
Gravy	Soups
Hard sauces	Waffles

A Special Note About Milk

Milk contains more than 25 different proteins, any one of which can induce an allergic reaction. Sometimes these various proteins are separated and used in the manufacturing of other products. For example, some foods labeled non-dairy contain casein, a milk protein. Be sure to read the labels. Butter is generally okay to use in moderate quantities. Margarine should not be used as it often contains milk proteins.

Foods That May Contain Eggs

Baking powder	Meringues
Batters used in frying	Noodles
Bouillon	Pancakes
Bread	Pasta
Cakes	Pretzels
Cookies	Pudding
French toast	Rolls
Fritters	Salad dressing
Frostings	Sauces
Hollandaise sauce	Sausage
Ice cream	Sherbets
Macaroni	Soufflés
Marshmallows	Soups
Meat loaf	Spaghetti
Meat patties	Waffles

Foods That May Contain Corn

Baking mixes	Grape juice
Batters used in frying	Gravy
Beer	Grits

Bleached wheat flour
Breads and pastries
Cakes
Candy
Carbonated beverages
Cheeses
Chewing gum
Chili
Chips
Chop suey
Cookies
Corn flakes and other cereals
Corn syrup
Corn starch
French dressing
Frostings
Gelatin desserts
Graham crackers

Hominy
Ice cream
Jams
Jellies
Ketchup
Margarine
Meat
Bacon
Bologna
Cold cuts
Frankfurters
Ham
Sausages
Peanut butter
Pies, cream
Puddings
Tortilla chips

Resources

There are many doctors located throughout the United States and Canada who are qualified to help with your allergies and allergy-related health problems. To find one of these doctors, contact one of the groups listed below for a referral. These doctors have all been trained in specific adjustment techniques that help balance body systems. They deal with chronic health problems including allergy, and will counsel you toward a healthier lifestyle.

Association of Naturopathic Physicians of British Columbia
#204 - 2786 West 16th Avenue
Vancouver, British Columbia V6K 3C4
(604) 732-7070

Bio-Energetic Synchronization Technique
1000 West Poplar, Suite "B"
Rogers, Arkansas 72751
1 (800) 874-1478 or (501) 631-2749
* Originated by Dr. M.T. Morter Jr.

International College of Applied Kinesiology
114 East 1823 Road
Lawrence, Kansas 66046-9236
(913) 542-1801
*(Founded by Dr. George Goodheart)

Neuro-Emotional Technique
500 Second Street
Encinitas, California 92024
(619) 753-1533
*(Originated by Dr. Scott Walker)

Ontario Naturopathic Medicine Association
60 Berl Avenue
Toronto, Ontario M8Y 3C7
(416) 503-9554

Total Body Modification
1907 E. Foxmore Circle
Sandy, Utah 84092
1 (801) 243-4TBM or 1 (801) 571-2411
* A total body technique originated by Dr. Victor Frank

Works Cited

Aihara, Herman. *Acid and Alkaline.* Oroville, California: George Oshawa Macrobiotic Foundation, 1986.

Allergy Foundation of America. *Allergy Its Mysterious Causes and Modern Treatment.* New York: Grosset & Dunlap, 1967.

Appleton, Nancy, PhD. *Healthy Bones.* Garden City Park, New York: Avery Publishing Group Inc., 1991.

Appleton, Nancy, PhD. *Lick The Sugar Habit.* Garden City Park, New York: Avery Publishing Group Inc., 1988.

Atkins, Robert C., MD. *Dr. Atkins' Health Revolution.* New York: Bantam Books, 1990.

Balch, James F., MD, and Balch, Phyllis A., CNC. *Prescription for Nutritional Healing.* Garden City Park, New York: Avery Publishing Group Inc., 1990.

Becker, Robert O., MD, and Marino, Andrew A., PhD. *Electromagnetism and Life.* Albany, New York: State University of New York Press, 1982.

Becker, Robert O., MD, and Selden, Gary. *The Body Electric.* New York, NY: William Morrow and Company, Inc., 1985.

Becker, Robert O., MD. *Cross Currents.* Los Angelos, California: Jeremy P. Tarcher, Inc., 1990.

Behrman, Richard E., MD, and Vaughan, Victor C. III, MD. *Nelson Textbook of Pediatrics.* Philadelphia, PA: W.B. Saunders Company, 1987.

Berkson, Lindsey D. *Healthy Digestion the Natural Way,* New York, New York: John Wiley & Sons, Inc., 2000.

Bierman, C. Warren, MD, and Pierson, William E., MD. "Disease of the ear." *Journal of Allergy and Immunology.* 81 (May 1988) 1009-1014.

Bland, Jeffrey, PhD. *Digestive Enzymes.* New Canaan, Connecticut: Keats Publishing, Inc., 1983.

Blaylock, Russell L. *Excitotoxins: the Taste That Kills,* Santa Fe, New Mexico; Health Press, 1994.

Bluestone, Charles D., MD, and Doyle, William J., PhD. "Anatomy and physiology of Eustachian tube and middle ear related to otitis media." *Journal of Allergy and Clinical Immunology.* 81 (May, 1988) 1004-1009.

Bottomley, H.W., MD, FACP. *Allergy; Its Treatment and Care.* New York: Funk & Wagnalls, 1968.

271

Braley, James, MD. Dr. Braly's *Food Allergy and Nutrition Revolution.* New Canaan, Connecticut; Keats Publishing, Inc., 1992.

Breneman, James C., MD. *Basics of Food Allergy.* Second Edition. Springfield, Illinois: Charles C. Thomas, Publisher, 1984.

Brostoff, Dr. Jonathan and Gamlin, Linda. *The Complete Guide to Food Allergy and Intolerance.* New York: Crown Publishers, Inc., 1989.

Brostoff, Jonathan, MA, DM, FRCP, and Chalacombe, Stephen JBDS, MRC. Path. *Food Allergy and Intolerance.* London, England: Bailliere Tindall, 1987.

Budwig, Dr. Johanna. *Flax Oil as a True Aid Against Arthritis, Heart Infarction, Cancer and Other Diseases.* Vancouver, British Columbia: Apple Publishing Company, 1992.

Buist, Robert, PhD. *Food Chemical Sensitivity.* Garden City Park, New York; Avery Publishing Group, Inc., 1988.

Burr, Harold Saxton. *Blueprint for Immortality.* Saffron, Walden: The C.W. Daniel Company Limited, 1988.

Burton, Benjamin T., PhD, and Foster, Willis R., MD. *Human Nutrition.* New York: McGraw Hill Book Company, 1988.

Cheraskin, E., MD, DMD, Ringsdorf, W.M., Jr., DMD, and Clark, J.W., DDS. *Diet and Disease.* New Canaan, Connecticut: Keats Publishing, Inc., 1968.

Chiaramonte, Lawrence T., Schneider, Arlene T., and Lifshitz, Iiama (edited by). *Food Allergy.* New York, New York: Marcel Dekker, Inc., 1988.

Cichoke, Anthony J. DC. *The Complete Book of Enzyme Therapy,* Garden City Park, New York; Avery Publishing Group, 1999.

Cichoke, Anthony J. DC. *Enzymes and Enzyme Therapy.* New Canaan, Connecticut; Keats Publishing, 1994.

Cocoa, Arthur F., MD. *Familial Nonreagenic Food Allergy.* Springfield, Illinois: Charles C. Thomas, Publisher, 1953.

Crook, William G., MD. *The Yeast Connection.* Jackson, Tennessee: Professional Books, 1984.

Crook, William G., MD. *Help for the Hyperactive Child.* Jackson, Tennessee: Professional Books, 1991.

Cutler, Ellen W. DC. *The Food Allergy Cure.* New York, New York; Harmony Books, 2001.

Cutler, Ellen W. DC. *Winning the War against Asthma & Allergies.* Albany, New York; Delmar Publishers, 1998.

Cutler, Ellen W. DC. *Winning the War against Immune Disorders & Allergies.* Albany, New York; Delmar Publishers, 1998.

Day, Charlene A. *The Immune System Handbook.* North York, Ontario: Potentials Within, 1991.

Diamond, John, MD. *Your Body Doesn't Lie,* New York, New York; Harper & Row, Publishers Inc., 1979

Dickey, Lawrence D., MD, FACS, edited by. *Clinical Ecology.* Springfield, Illinois: Charles C. Thomas, Publisher, 1976.

Engel, June, PhD. *The Complete Allergy Book.* Toronto, Ontario; Key Porter Books LTD, 1997.

Erasmus, Udo. *Fats and Oils.* Vancouver, Canada: Alive Books, 1986.

Erasmus, Udo. *Fats That Heal, Fats That Kill.* Vancouver, Canada: Alive Books, 1993.

Fireman, Phillip, MD, and Slavin, Raymond G., MD. *Atlas of Allergies.* New York, New York: Gower Medical Publishing, 1991.

Gerber, Richard, MD. *Vibrational Medicine.* Santa Fe, New Mexico: Bear & Company, 1988.

Gittleman, Ann Louise. *Guess What Came To Dinner.* Garden city Park, New York; Avery Publishing Group inc., 1993.

Goldberger, Emanual, MD, FACP. *A Primer of Water, Electrolyte, and Acid-Base Syndromes,* 7th Edition. Philadelphia, PA: Lea & Febiger, 1986.

Gottschall, Elaine, BA, MSc. *Food and the Gut Reaction.* Kirkton, Ontario: The Kirkton Press, 1990.

Gottschall, Elaine, BA, MSc. *Breaking the Vicious Cycle.* Kirkton, Ontario, The Kirkton Press, 1994.

Gursche, Siegfried, MH. *Encyclopedia of Natural Healing.* Burnaby, BC; Alive Publishing, Inc., 1997.

Guyton, Arthur C., MD. *Textbook of Medical Physiology,* 7th Edition. Philadelphia, PA: W.B. Saunders Company, 1986.

Halperin, M.L., MD, and Goldstein, Marc B., MD. *Fluid Electrolyte, and Acid-Base Emergencies.* Philadelphia, PA: W.B. Saunders Company, 1988.

Halpern, Seymour L., MD, FACP, FACN. *Clinical Nutrition.* Philadelphia, PA: J.B. Lippincott Company, 1987.

Harris, M. Coleman, MD. *All About Allergy.* Englewood Cliffs, New Jersey: Prentice-Hall, Inc., 1969.

Howell, Dr. Edward *Enzyme Nutrition.* Wayne, New Jersey: Avery Publishing Group Inc., 1985.

Howell, Dr. Edward. *Food Enzymes for Health and Longevity.* Woodstock Valley, Connecticut: Omangod Press, 1980.

Hunt, Douglas, MD. *No More Cravings.* New York, New York.: Warner Books, Inc., 1987.

Igram, Cass, DO. *Who Needs Headaches?* Cedar Rapids, Iowa: Literary Visions Publishing, Inc.

Kamen, Betty, PhD. *Startling New Facts About Osteoporosis.* Novato, CA: Nutrition Encounter, Inc., 1989. Keats Publishing, Inc., 1994

Kroeger, Hanna. *Parasites: The Enemy Within.* Colorado; Hanna Kroeger Publications, 1991.

La Tourelle, Maggie. *Thorsons Introductory Guide to Kinesiology.* London, England; Harper-Collins Publishers, 1992.

Lahoz, S. Colet RN. MS. *Conquering Yeast Infections.* Lac. Raleigh, North Carolina; Pentland Press, Inc., 1996.

Lawlor, Glenn J., MD, and Fisher, Thomas J., MD, edited by. *Manual of Allergy and Immunology.* Boston/Toronto: Little, Brown and Company, 1988.

Lee, Lita, Ph.D. *Radiation Protection Manual.* Sacramento, CA: Spilman Printing, 1990.

Lehninger, Albert L. *Principles of Biochemistry.* New York, New York: Worth Publishers, Inc., 1982

Linder, Maria C., PhD. *Nutritional Biochemistry and Metabolism.* New York, New York: Elsevier Science Publishing Company, Inc., 1985.

Lininger, Skye DC., Wright, Johathan, MD., Austin, Steve ND., Brown, Donald ND., Gaby, Alan MD. *The Natural Pharmacy.* Rocklin, California; Prima Publsihing, 1998.

Lipski, Elizabeth, MS, CCN. *Digestive Wellness.* New Canaan, Connecticut; Keats Publishing, Inc., 1996.

Lipski, Elizabeth, MS, CCN. *Leaky Gut Syndrome.* New Canaan, Connecticut; Keats Publishing, Inc., 1998.

Loomis, Howard F. Jr., DC, FIACA. *Enzymes The Key to Health.* Madison, WI; Grote Publishing, 1999.

Loomis, Howard F. Jr., DC. *Applied Patho-Physiology and Enzyme Nutrition.* Forsyth, MI: 21st Century Nutrition, Inc., 1990

Mandell, Dr. Marshall, and Scanlon, Lynne Waller. *Dr. Mandells 5-Day Allergy Relief System.* New York: Pocket Books, 1980.

Martens, Richard A., MD, and Martens, Sherlyn, MS, RD. *The Milk Sugar Dilemma: Living with Lactose Intolerance.* East Lansing, MI: Medi-Ed Press, 1967.

McDougall, John A., MD, and McDougall, Mary A. *The McDougall Plan.* Piscataway, NJ: New Century Publishers, 1983.

McKenna, John MD. Natural Alternatives to Antibiotics. Garden City Park, New York; Avery Publishing Group, 1998.

Miller, Martha J., MAT. *Pathophysiology Principles of Disease.* Philadelphia, PA: W.B. Saunders Co., 1983.

Moore, Richard, MD, PhD, and Webb, George D., PhD. *The K Factor.* New York, New York: Pocket Books, 1987.

Morell, Franz, MD. *The Mora Concept.* Heidelberg, Germany: Karl F. Haug Publishers, 1990.

Morter, M.T. Jr., BS, MA, DC. *Correlative Urinalysis.* Rogers, Arkansas: B.E.S.T. Research Inc., 1987.

Morter, Dr. M. Ted Jr. *Your Health Your Choice.* Hollywood, Florida: Fell Publishers, Inc., 1990.

Morter, M.T. Jr., BS, MA, DC. *The Healing Field.* Rogers, Arkansas: B.E.S.T. Research, Inc., 1991.

National Research Council. *Recommended Dietary Allowances, 10th edition.* Washington, DC: National Academy Press, 1989.

Paterson, Barbara. *The Allergy Connection.* Wellingborough, New York: Thorsons Publishers, Ltd., 1985. Penguin Books Ltd., 1996.

Patterson, Ray, MD. *Allergic Diseases.* Philadelphia, PA: J.B. Lippincott Company, 1972.

Pennington, Jean A.T., PhD, RD. *Food Values of Portions Commonly Used.* New York, New York: Harper & Row Publishers, Inc. 1989.

Pert, Candace B. PhD. *Molecules of Emotion.* New York, New York,; Touchstone, 1999.

Philpott, William H., MD, and Kalita, Dwight K., PhD. *Brain Allergies.* New Canaan, Connecticut: Keats Publishing, Inc., 1980.

Philpott, William H., MD, and Kalita, Dwight K., PhD. *Victory Over Diabetes.* New Canaan, Connecticut: Keats Publishing, Inc., 1983.

Pottenger, Francis M. Jr., MD. *Pottenger's Cats.* La Mesa, California: Price-Pottenger Nutrition Foundation, 1989.

Randolph, Theron G., MD, and Moss, Ralph W., PhD. *An Alternate Approach to Allergies.* New York: Harper & Row, Publishers, 1990.

Rapp, Doris J., MD. *Is This Your Child?* New York, New York; William Morrow and Company, Inc., 1991.

Rapp, Doris J., MD. *Allergies and Your Family.* New York: Sterling Publishing Co., Inc., 1985.

Roberts, H. J., MD. *Aspartame (NutraSweet)Is It Safe?* Philadelphia, Pennsylvania: The Charles Press, Publishers, 1990.

Roberts, Ron, and Sammut, Judy. *Asthma an Alternative Approach.* London, United Kingdom, Souvenir Press, 2000.

Rochlitz, Steven. *Allergies and Candida.* Mahopac, New York: Human Ecology Balancing Sciences, Inc., 1991.

Rona, Zoltan P. MD. *Childhood Illness and the Allergy Connection.* Rocklin, California; Prima Publishing, 1997.

Rona, Zoltan P. MD, MSc. *The Joy of Health.* Willowdale, Ontario; Hounslow Press, 1991.

Rona, Zoltan P. MD, MSc., *Return to the Joy of Health.* Burnaby BC; Alive Books, 1995.

Rowe, Albert H., MD. *Food Allergy.* Springfield, Illinois: Charles C. Thomas, Publisher, 1972.

Rubin, Emanuel, MD, and Farber, John L. MD. *Pathology.* Philadelphia, PA: J.B. Lippincott Company, 1988.

Sampson, Hugh A., MD, and Cooke, Sarak., S.B. "Food allergy and the potential allergenicity-antigenicity of microparticulated egg and cow's milk proteins." *Journal of the American College of Nutrition.* Vol. 9, No. 4, 410-417 (1990).

Santillo, Humbart, BS, MH. *Food Enzymes.* Prescott Valley, Arizona: Hohm Press, 1987.

Sargeant, Doris and Evans, Karen. *Hard to Swallow.* Burnaby, BC; Alive Books, 1999.

Schechter, Steven R., ND. *Fighting Radiation and Chemical Pollutants with Foods, Herbs, and Vitamins.* Encinitas, California: Vitality Link, 1990.

Schmidt, Michael A. *Childhood Ear Infections.* Berkeley, California: North Atlantic Books, 1990.

Schwarz, Edward F., PhD. *Endocrines, Organs, and their Impact.* Hales Corners, WI: Cornerstone Press, 1985.

Seldin & Giebish. *The Regulation of Acid-Base Balance.* New York: Raven Press, Ltd., 1989.

Sheinkin, David, MD, Schachter, Michael, MD, and Hutton, Richard. *The Food Connection.* Indianapolis/New York: The Bobbs-Merrill Company, Inc., 1979.

Speer, Frederic, MD. *Food Allergy.* New York: John Wright PSE. Inc., 1983.

Stone, Robert B., PhD. *The Secret Life of Your Cells.* Westchester, PA.: Whitford Press, 1989.

Szekely, Edmond Bordeaux *The Essene Gospel of Peace.* United States: International Biogenic Society, 1981.

Taube, E. Louis, MD. *Food Allergy and the Allergic Patient.* Springfield, Illinois: Charles C. Thomas, Publisher, 1978.

Thompson, W. Grant, MD. *Gut Reactions.* New York/London: Plenum Press, 1989.

Trowbridge, John Parkes, MD, and Walker, Morton, DPM. *The Yeast Syndrome.* Toronto/New York: Bantam Books, 1986.

Truss, C. Orion, MD. *The Missing Diagnosis.* Birmingham, Alabama; Published by C. Orion Truss, 1986.

Valentine, Bob and Carole and Hetrick, Douglas P., DC. *Applied Kinesiology.* Rochester, New York; Healing Arts Press, 1987.

Vanderhaeghe, Lorna R. and Bouic, Patrick J.D, PhD. *The Immune System Cure.* Scarborough, Ontario; Prentice-Hall Canada, Inc., 1999.

Washton, Arnold, PhD, and Boundy, Donna, MSW. *Willpower's Not Enough.* New York: Harper Collins, Publishers, 1990.

Weintraub, Sky ND. *The Parasite Menace.* Pleasant Grove, Utah; Woodland Publishing, 1998.

Werbach, Melvyn, R., MD. *Nutritional Influences on Illness.* Tarzana, California: Third Line Press, Inc., 1988.

Werbach, Melvyn, R., MD. *Third Line Medicine.* Guernsey, Channel Islands: The Guernsey Press Co. Ltd., 1986.

Williams, Warwick, Dyson, Bannister. *Gray's Anatomy.* Thirty-Seventh Edition. Edinburgh, London: Churchill Livingstone, 1989.

Wolf, Max, MD, and Ransberger, Karl, PhD. *Enzyme Therapy.* Los Angeles, California: Regent House, 1977.

Zimmerman, Barry, MD., Gold, Milton, MD., Lavi, Sasson, MD., Feanny, Stephen, MD. *The Canadian Allergy and Asthma Handbook.* Mississauga, Ontario; Random House of Canada Limited, 1991.

Index

friendly, 106–108
Balance, 27
Barberry root bark, 96
Base-acid balance, 141
Beasley, Joseph D., 98
Becker, Robert O., MD, 223, 225, 230
Bed wetting, 45, 192-195
Beer, 79
Belching, 45
Benzoic acid and sodium benzoate, 214
BHA and BHT, 209
Bile, 101
Biochemical individuality, 15
Black walnut, 96
Blackouts, 44
Bladder infection, 72
Blastocystis hominis, 93
Blastomyces, 82
Bleeding, 45
  gums, 170
Bloating, 45, 72, 88, 97, 138
Blood
  cells, white, 54, 61, 122-123
  in stool, 88
  pH, 104
  pressure, high, 44
  test for parasites, 86
  vessels, 48
Bowel disease, inflammatory, 68, 88
Brain waves, 224
Braly, James, MD, 104, 206
Bread and rolls, 169
Breastfeeding, 188-189
Breath, shortness of, 67, 68
Breneman, Dr. James C., 50, 180, 193
Brittle nails, 170
Bronchitis, 44
Bruising, 45
Bueno, Dr. Hermann R., 84
Burr, Harold Saxton, 224

C

Cabbage, 101

Caesar dressing, recipe, 177
Calcium, 119, 155
  myths, 157-159
  non-dairy sources of, 160-162
  supplements, 158–159
Cancer, 92, 127
Canned meat, 123
Candida albicans, 71, 79, 189
  diet, 239-241
  reduction program, 238-239
Candidiasis, 72
  and allergy, 76-78
  and parasites, 83
  diagnosing, 76
  factors leading to, 74
  symptoms of, 75-76
Candy, 169
Canker sores, 45
Canola oil, 171
Car exhaust, 72
Carbonated beverages, 123, 155
Cat studies, Pottenger, 130, 235
Cataracts, 45
Causes of allergy, 32
Cells
  in allergic state, 151, 154
  in normal state, 153
Cellular phone, 233
Cellulase, 121
Cheese, 79
Chemical
  allergies, 205-216
  sensitivity and intolerance, 67, 68, 76, 231
Chest pain, 44, 231, see also Angina and Heartburn
Chewing, 117
Childhood conditions, 180-203
Chiropractic adjustment, 201, 245
Chocolate, 103, 155
Cholesterol, 163
Cinnamon, 193
Circulatory symptoms of allergy, 44
Citrus bioflavonoids, 250
Cloves, 96
Coffee, 103

About the Author

Dr. Carolee Bateson-Koch completed her basic science requirements at Fresno State College in California before entering the Los Angeles College of Chiropractic. She received her Doctor of Chiropractic degree in 968, graduating as valedictorian of her class. Dr. Bateson-Koch continued postgraduate studies, earning a PhD in nutrition.

In 1988, she received her Doctor of Naturopathy degree from the Ontario College of Naturopathy in Canada and was honored with the nutrition award for her graduating class.

Dr. Bateson-Koch lectures internationally and has appeared on numerous television and radio shows throughout North America. She is the author of many articles on health and is a contributing author to the *Encyclopedia of Natural Healing*.

Dr. Bateson-Koch has traveled throughout the United States, Canada, China, Germany and Australia gathering information on safe and useful therapies for allergy.

Many thanks to:
The staff at Alive Books who have been so helpful.

Book Publishing Co.

Community owned since 1974

books that educate, inspire, and empower

To find your favorite vegetarian and soyfood products online, visit:

www.healthy-eating.com

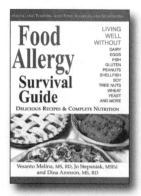

Food Allergy Survival Guide
Vesanto Melina, MS,RD,
Jo Stepaniak, MSEd,
Dina Aronson, RD
978-1-57067-163-0 $19.95

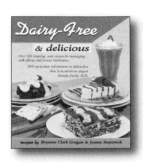

Dairy-Free & Delicious
Bryanna Clark Grogan,
Jo Stepaniak
978-1-57067-124-1 $14.95

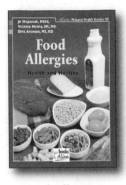

Food Allergies
Vesanto Melina, MS, RD,
Jo Stepaniak, MSEd,
Dina Aronson, RD
978-1-55321-046-9 $11.95

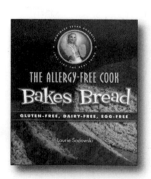

The Allergy-Free Cook Bakes Bread
Laurie Sadowski
978-1-57067-262-0 $14.95

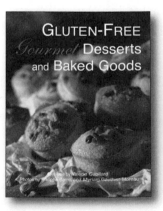

Gluten-Free Gourmet Desserts and Baked Goods
Valérie Cupillard
978-1-57067-187-6 $24.95

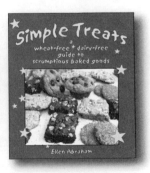

Simple Treats
Ellen Abraham
978-1-57067-137-1 $14.95

Purchase these health titles and cookbooks from your local bookstore or
natural food store, or you can buy them directly from:

Book Publishing Company • P.O. Box 99 • Summertown, TN 38483
1-800-695-2241

Please include $3.95 per book for shipping and handling.

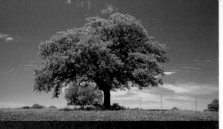

allergies

Disease in Disguise

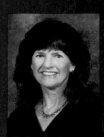

Carolee Bateson-Koch is a doctor of chiropractic and naturopathy with a special interest in the treatment of allergic conditions using natural therapies and nutrition. She has successfully treated hundreds of patients. Drawing on 25 years of clinical experience and information gathered from travels throughout the United States, Canada, China, Germany and Australia, she lectures and writes to increase professional and public awareness of the scope of allergic diseases and their effective treatment.

$15.95 US
$18.95 Canada

Learn to identify your symptoms and get well using proven, innovative, drug-free therapies

Allergy is generally misunderstood. It can show up as almost any symptom, but is rarely diagnosed. Left untreated it can lead to serious degenerative disease. Asthma, migraines, arthritis, ulcers and obesity have all been linked to allergy. Fatigue, irritability, body aching, digestive problems and other vague ailments are typical of allergy.

Allergies: Disease in Disguise is the first book ever to explain how to achieve complete and permanent recovery. Drugs may relieve or manage symptoms but will never make a person well. Alternative, healthful treatments, based on an understanding of what allergy is and how it works in the body, can heal the underlying allergic condition so that no further treatment of any kind is required.

Dr. Bateson-Koch provides insight into why allergy is becoming more common, how it relates to environmental factors, food additives, diet, digestion, body chemistry, addiction, yeasts, molds, parasites and childhood illnesses – and why enzymes are the key to healing.

Following her program, you won't have to give up your pet, get allergy shots, rotate foods, keep diet diaries or cook allergy-free recipes for the rest of your life. You will not only recover and enjoy an allergy-free life, you will gain invaluable understanding of health and well-being.

books Alive

ISBN 978-1-55312-040-7